The **First-aid** Handbook

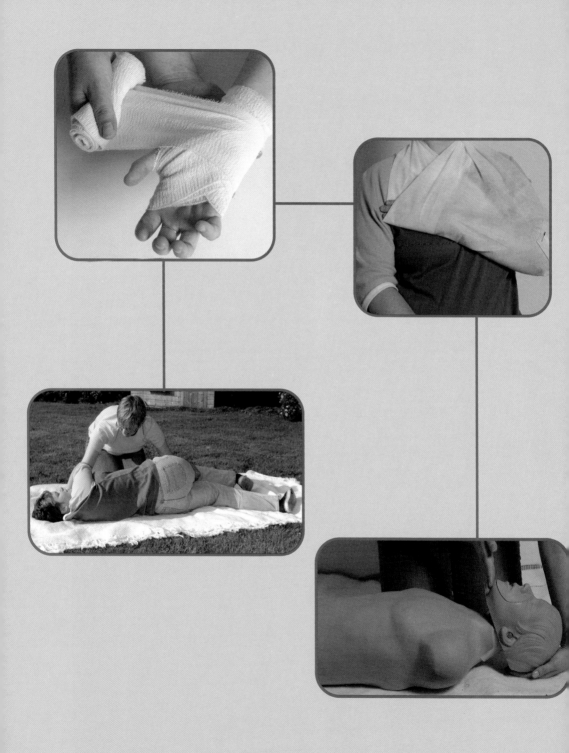

The **First-aid** **Handbook**

Maria Costantino

Published by

SILVERDALE BOOKS

An imprint of Bookmart Ltd
Registered number 2372865
Trading as Bookmart Ltd
Desford Road
Enderby
Leicester LE19 4AD

@ 2003 D&S Books Ltd

D&S Books Ltd
Kerswell,
Parkham Ash, Bideford
Devon, England
EX39 5PR

e-mail us at:-
enquiries@dsbooks.fsnet.co.uk

This edition printed 2003

ISBN 1-856057-34-8

Creative Director: Sarah King
Editor: Clare Haworth-Maden
Project Editor: Anna Southgate
Photographer: Paul Forrester/Colin Bowling
Designer: Axis Design

Fonts used: Arial Rounded; Gadget

Printed in China

1 3 5 7 9 10 8 6 4 2

Contents

Introduction

Immediate action is necessary in an emergency, and is often the most valuable help that can be given. First aid is the first assistance or treatment that is administered when someone suffers an injury or suddenly becomes ill. From minor injuries to major emergencies, a working knowledge of first-aid practice can limit the distress suffered, and injuries sustained, by a casualty, and in some instances can actually save someone's life.

An inexperienced first-aider can, however, often feel at a loss when it comes to knowing what to do in an emergency. In many cases, the patient's injuries or illness will be minor, requiring only common sense and some basic treatment to ensure that he or she is calmed down and made comfortable. In such circumstances, even the most inexperienced first-aiders are doing a good job if they stay calm and are sympathetic and reassuring.

Although this book is designed to help the first-aider to deal with urgent situations when no other help is readily available, a full first-aid training course is highly recommended for everyone. The life-saving techniques of artificial respiration (AR) and cardiopulmonary resuscitation (CPR) are explained, but it is vital that these procedures are studied under a qualified instructor and using an approved training manikin. AR and CPR techniques can be mastered by everyone, but they are skills for which practice is essential. Learning first aid with a qualified instructor will give you the knowledge and confidence to be able to act quickly, calmly, confidently and effectively in an emergency – a situation that could mean the difference between life and death. You will find details of the organisations that run first-aid training courses at the back of this book (see page 256).

Introduction

What to do before an emergency happens

Don't wait for an accident or emergency to happen before preparing yourself. Read the information in this book carefully and also observe the following points.

· Take a first-aid course led by a qualified instructor. No book can ever be a substitute for a good-quality training course.

· Learn how to administer AR and CPR. Knowing these life-saving techniques can mean the difference between life and death.

· Make sure that you have a well-stocked first-aid kit at home, in your car, caravan or boat, as well as in your suitcase when you go on holiday.

· Make sure that you and your children know how to ask for help from the emergency services. Teach your children how to use the telephone correctly, how to dial emergency numbers and how to listen to instructions. Ensure, too, that you know how to telephone for help when you are in a foreign country.

Calling the emergency services

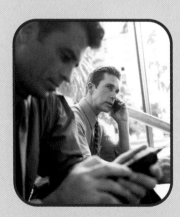

You can call the emergency services – the police, fire brigade and ambulance service – free of charge from home telephones, public call boxes and mobile phones.

In areas such as national parks, mountainous regions and by rivers and the sea, further emergency services, such as forest rangers, mountain rescue, inshore and offshore lifeboats and coast guards, will also be available.

If you have a mobile phone, make sure that the battery is always fully charged. Be warned that mobile phones may not operate in certain areas, in which case you will need to use a land line for emergency calls.

Before calling the emergency services, follow these guidelines.

· Whenever possible, stay with the casualty, send someone else to phone for assistance and ask them to return to you to confirm that the call has been made.

· If you are the only person present in an emergency, and help is unlikely to arrive, seek aid as soon as possible.

· Call 999 (in the UK), 911 (in the USA) or 000 (in Australian state capitals; telephone directories will list any alternative numbers) and ask for the most appropriate service. The emergency operator will contact and advise other emergency services if they are required.

Note that you must provide the following information clearly and calmly.

· The number from which you are calling so that the emergency services can contact you again if they need to.

· The location or address at which the accident or incident occurred. If you know them, give local road names, postal districts or areas, along with the proximity to road junctions or any conspicuous buildings or landmarks.

· The nature of the incident, the number of people injured, as well as their age and sex, and the type of injuries that they have sustained.

· Whether there are any hazards that you know about, such as leaking gas, petroleum or chemical spills, damaged power lines or live electrical cables.

Finally, do not hang up the receiver until the emergency control operator tells you to do so.

Introduction

What to do in an emergency

In an emergency, remember that the aims of first aid are:
· to preserve life;
· to prevent a casualty's injuries worsening;
· to aid recovery.

More specifically, the first-aider's tasks are:
· to ascertain what has happened;
· to be aware of any dangers and to deal with them appropriately;
· to act calmly and efficiently in dealing with an injury or illness;
· to arrange the next stage of the patient's care. This may mean making sure that the patient can get home, advising him or her to consult a doctor or organising transportation to the hospital.

Apart from calling the emergency services, there are a number of things that you should – and shouldn't – do in an emergency, such as a road accident.

· Do not approach a casualty unless it is safe to do so. Before doing so, check whether there is any danger to you, to others or to the injured person.

· When confronted by a road accident, make the accident scene safe. Position red warning triangles 200 metres (220 yards) away in both directions. Park your vehicle so that it blocks off any oncoming traffic and switch on your hazard-warning lights. Check under any debris inside the vehicles involved to ascertain whether any casualties are hidden from view.

· Do not try to move a casualty trapped inside a vehicle unless he or she is in immediate danger from fire or an adequate airway (see pages 38 to 40) cannot be maintained.

· Do not smash a vehicle's windscreen or window unless the casualty will be protected from the broken glass.

· Do not attempt to right an overturned vehicle.

· Do not disconnect the battery of a damaged vehicle.

· Do not smoke, or allow anyone else to smoke, near a crashed vehicle.

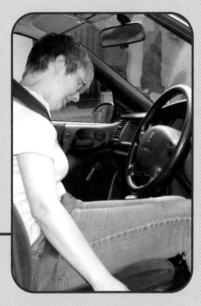

If a casualty in a road accident is not in immediate danger from fire, and an adequate airway can be maintained, do not move him or her.

Introduction

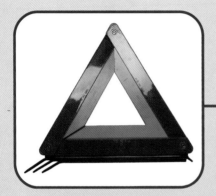

Red warning triangle.

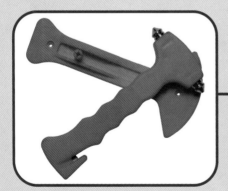

Safety hammer.

· Do not remove the helmets of injured motorcyclists or cyclists – leave this to the emergency services. If, however, it is vital that you administer artificial respiration (see pages 44 to 46), ask an assistant to support the casualty's head and neck and to keep them in line with the spine while the helmet's restraining straps are cut or undone and the helmet is very carefully eased over the top of the casualty's head. Again, however, do not remove a helmet unless it is a matter of life and death. (For more information, see pages 32 to 33.)

· Road accidents may be complicated by spillages of hazardous substances. Vans and trucks carrying chemicals or compressed and liquid gases display a warning panel indicating the substances that they are transporting, their properties, a special identifying code number and a telephone number. Make a careful note of this information to give to the emergency services when you contact them. It is vital that you do not approach a vehicle that is carrying toxic or hazardous substances.

· Do not attempt any rescue or treatment unless you are sure that you will not come into contact with a hazardous substance.

There are specific things to be aware of if the emergency involves electricity or fire.

· When a casualty is in contact with electricity, do not attempt first aid until the contact has been broken in case you electrocute yourself. The current must be stopped immediately, either by switching it off at the mains or by removing the appliance's plug. If this is impossible, you'll have to move the part of the casualty's body that is making contact with the electrical current. Do this by standing on a dry surface (such as a piece of wood, a folded newspaper or a rubber mat) and using a non-conductive material (a rolled-up newspaper or a wooden broom handle, for example) to knock that part of the casualty's body clear of the electrical current.

· If you are confronted by a fire, act quickly by calling the emergency services and giving them as much precise information as possible.

· Do not enter a smoke-filled building or room because there is a serious danger that you could be overcome by smoke or burnt.

· Do not attempt to extinguish a big fire, but instead call the emergency services.

. If you are trapped in a room, shut the door and open a window. If it is possible to escape through a window, don't jump, but instead carefully lower yourself to the ground, feet first. If escape is not possible, wait for the emergency services to rescue you.

· If someone is on fire, use the stop, drop, wrap and roll procedure described on page 110.

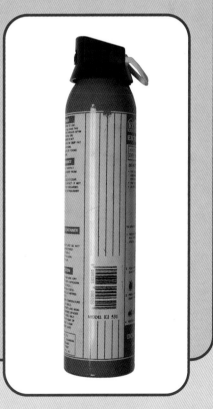

Fire extinguisher.

Introduction

Here are some final first-aid tips to remember if you find yourself in an emergency situation.

· Do not attempt to do too much! Good first-aiders know that ambulance paramedics are far more knowledgeable than they are, so only administer essential first aid.

· Do treat the most serious conditions and injuries first, and always watch for signs of shock (see pages 92 to 94).

· Do not try to make a precise diagnosis – this will be made by a doctor once the casualty has been admitted to hospital. Do, however, look for signs and symptoms of injuries, such as bleeding, bruising, swelling or deformed limbs.

· Do not move a casualty unless it is absolutely essential to do so for safety reasons. (For guidelines on moving a casualty, see pages 22 to 31.)

· Do not leave a casualty alone, but instead send someone else for help. If you are the only person present in an emergency, and help is unlikely to arrive, however, seek help as soon as possible.

· Do not give a casualty anything to eat or drink, but do keep them warm and as comfortable as possible, and constantly offer them reassurance.

Avoiding cross-infection

It is nowadays necessary to assume that an injured and bleeding casualty may be infected by certain viruses, such as human immunodeficiency virus (HIV) and Hepatitis B and Hepatitis C, which are transmitted by blood-to-blood contact. As a first-aider, if you have a cut, puncture, sore or other type of open wound, you therefore risk infection when treating an injured person.

Although it is important to note that the risk of infection is very small – much smaller than is commonly imagined – you must always take certain elementary precautions.

· Always assume spilled blood and other bodily fluids to be infected.
· Wash away any of the casualty's blood that has come into contact with your skin as soon as possible. Remember, however, that the risk of becoming infected in this way is very small.
· Whenever possible, wash your hands thoroughly both before and after treating a casualty, making sure that you wash both the fronts and the backs of your hands.

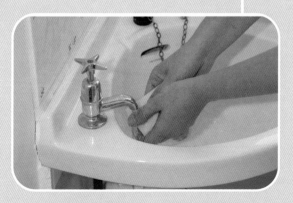

Wherever possible, wash your hands before and after administering first aid.

· Avoid getting a casualty's blood in your eyes. Although the risk is, again, small, infection can occur via the conjunctiva.

· The risk from saliva contamination during mouth-to-mouth artificial respiration is believed to be negligible. If, however, there is bleeding in, or around, a casualty's mouth, or from other facial injuries, which does pose a risk, you can avoid skin-to-skin contact by placing a thin plastic bag with a slit cut in it over the casualty's mouth and then performing AR by blowing through the slit. Or you can use a face shield if your first-aid kit contains one.

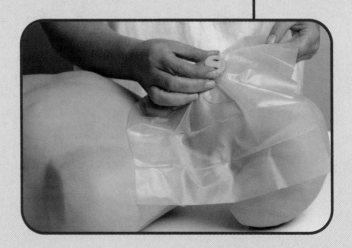

· If they are available, wear disposable gloves before coming into contact with blood or applying or disposing of sterile dressings. If no gloves are available, improvise by covering your hands with clean plastic bags.

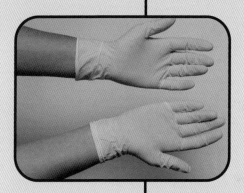

· Dispose of first-aid waste carefully. For hypodermic needles and syringes, use yellow 'sharps' containers, which are special containers designed for the secure disposal of sharp implements that are collected and disposed of safely by authorised waste-removal operatives. Specially marked yellow plastic bags are also available for disposing of soiled dressings, which are then sealed and incinerated.

Introduction

Chapter 1

Emergency priorities, actions and techniques

In an emergency, you need to prioritise your actions and then act quickly, calmly and efficiently. If he or she is unconscious, the person's life may be in danger: the airway may be blocked, breathing may have stopped and blood circulation may have ceased. You will need to act quickly in such a situation because brain damage or death may result.

Step-by-step emergency action plan

Step 1 Assess the scene

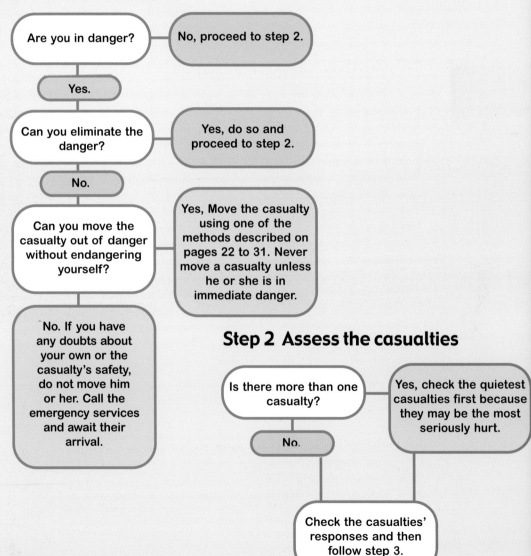

Are you in danger?

No, proceed to step 2.

Yes.

Can you eliminate the danger?

Yes, do so and proceed to step 2.

No.

Can you move the casualty out of danger without endangering yourself?

Yes, Move the casualty using one of the methods described on pages 22 to 31. Never move a casualty unless he or she is in immediate danger.

No. If you have any doubts about your own or the casualty's safety, do not move him or her. Call the emergency services and await their arrival.

Step 2 Assess the casualties

Is there more than one casualty?

Yes, check the quietest casualties first because they may be the most seriously hurt.

No.

Check the casualties' responses and then follow step 3.

Step 3 Emergency procedure

Check whether the casualty is conscious or unconscious.

If unconscious, turn onto their side in the recovery position. Check the airway and clear it if necessary.

If conscious, treat serious conditions, such as major bleeding; treat for shock if required, treat minor injuries.

Make comfortable and hand over to the emergency services.

Check breathing.

If not breathing begin artificial respiration (AR).

If breathing, leave in the recovery position; check the airway, breathing and circulation (pulse) frequently.

After giving five full breaths in ten seconds of AR, check the pulse.

Check for injuries; stop any bleeding; treat for shock if required.

If pulse is present, continue AR at fifteen breaths a minute. Check breathing every two minutes until help arrives.

If there is no pulse, begin cardiopulmonary resuscitation (CPR). Check breathing and pulse every two minutes. Continue with CPR until help arrives.

Make comfortable and hand over to the emergency services.

Emergency priorities, actions and techniques

Moving and lifting casualties

The first-aider's first consideration should be the casualty's well-being, and the casualty's condition must not be aggravated, or his or her life endangered, by careless handling. Never move an injured person unless there is a serious threat to his or her life, for example, if a building is on fire, in danger of collapse or is filling up with gas or poisonous fumes, such as carbon monoxide.

Before moving a casualty

Avoid moving anyone with severe crush injuries because this could cause greater damage.

If it is absolutely necessary to move a casualty, first assess the nature and severity of the injuries, especially to the neck or spine. Examine the casualty's head and neck, chest and abdomen, as well as all of the limbs. The limbs must be supported while they are being moved, especially if the casualty is unconscious, so before beginning, support the joints above and below any suspected fracture or any other type of serious injury. Never attempt to move a casualty on your own if help is available, and instead ask for assistance.

If you are unsure about the exact nature and severity of a casualty's injuries, but he or she is conscious and breathing freely, try to keep the casualty in precisely the same position in which he or she was found during the moving process.

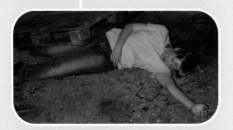

Avoid moving a casualty with crush injuries.

Moving and lifting a casualty

1 Get as close to the casualty as possible.

2 Spread your feet at a comfortable distance to ensure that you are stable and balanced.

3 Lower yourself to the level of the casualty by bending your knees. Never bend your back, but instead keep it straight.

4 Grasp the casualty firmly, using every part of your hands.

5 Lift the casualty by drawing on the strength of your legs, not your back, and using your shoulders to bear the casualty's weight.

6 Should the casualty begin to slip, let him or her slide gently to the ground. This will prevent the casualty from being injured further and will also avoid you injuring your back.

7 Remember that you should never try to lift too heavy a weight on your own. Get help whenever possible because the greater the number of people lifting a casualty, the lower the risk of causing or incurring an injury.

Moving and lifting methods

There are a number of methods that can be used to move and lift casualties, with the most suitable method depending on a number of factors:

· the size and weight of the injured person;

· the number of helpers available;

· the distance that the casualty needs to be moved and the terrain over which he or she has to be carried;

· the type and severity of the injuries sustained;

· the available equipment.

Emergency priorities, actions and techniques

Moving a casualty: one first-aider

These methods should only be used by a solitary first-aider when a casualty cannot be lifted, or is not capable of standing up, and needs to be removed from further danger very quickly. Avoid using any of these methods if you suspect that the casualty has sustained neck or head injuries.

1.1

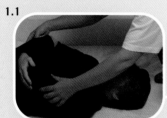

1.2

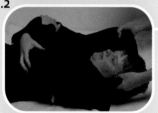

Dragging method 1.

Dragging method 1
1 If he or she is wearing one, unbutton the casualty's jacket or overcoat and then fold the casualty's arms across his or her chest.
2 Pull back the jacket or overcoat and place it underneath the person's head.
3 Bending your knees, crouch down behind the casualty's head, firmly grasp the jacket or coat's shoulders and then tug the casualty away.

2

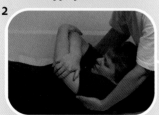

Dragging method 2.

Dragging method 2
1 Fold one of the casualty's arms across his or her chest.
2 Slide your arms beneath the casualty's armpits and then firmly grasp both arms.
3 Cradling the person's head in your arms, gently drag the casualty away. If possible, ask someone to help you to keep the casualty's head and body in line as you are dragging him or her away.

Dragging method 3
Only use this method if the casualty is not wearing a jacket or coat, unlike in method 1.
1 Fold the casualty's arms across his or her chest.
2 Crouch down behind the casualty's head and slide your hands underneath the person's armpits.
3 Cradling his or her head in your arms, gently drag the person away.

Dragging method 4
This method can be used either to drag a very heavy casualty or to move a person some distance away from imminent danger.
1 Cross the casualty's arms at the wrists.
2 Using a belt or scarf, tie the casualty's wrists together. Wind the material around the wrists tightly, but not so tightly that it impedes circulation. Tie the ends with a reef knot (see page 73) and then quickly check that the knot is secure.
3 Kneel down astride the casualty and slip your head through his or her bound wrists so that they are resting on your shoulders at the base of your neck.
4 Push yourself up into a crouch and then drag the casualty forwards, using your arms to take the weight and keeping the casualty's head clear of the ground.

Emergency priorities, actions and techniques

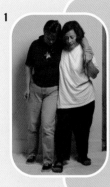

The human crutch

Use the human crutch when the casualty is conscious and is able to stand and walk with assistance – if he or she has a sprained ankle, for example.

1 Stand close to the casualty's injured side (unless the injury is to the hand, arm or shoulder, in which case you should support the uninjured side). Put your arm around the casualty's waist and grip his or her clothing at the hip.

2 Ask the person to put an arm around your neck and then take hold of that hand.

3 Supporting the casualty's weight with your body, move forward using small, slow steps, taking the first step together with the inside foot.

The piggyback ride

Use the piggyback ride if the casualty is conscious and a lightweight person or child who is strong enough to hold onto you.

The cradle

The cradle is another method whereby the solitary first-aider can carry a child or lightweight casualty: simply position one arm under the thighs and the other above the person's waist.

The fireman's lift 1

This method can be used to carry a conscious or unconscious lightweight adult or child away from danger, at the same time enabling the first-aider to keep one hand free.

1 Help the casualty to stand up and then grasp his or her right wrist with your left hand.

2 With one foot positioned a little in front of the other and your knees bent, lean forwards, gently place your right shoulder into the casualty's groin area and let the person fall gently across your shoulders.

3 Place your right arm around the back of the casualty's knees.

4 Raise yourself to a standing position, adjusting the casualty's weight across your shoulders.

The fireman's lift 2

This fireman's-lift method can be used when the casualty is unable to stand.

1 Turn the casualty so that he or she is lying face downwards. Facing the casualty, bend your knees and drop into a squatting position.

2 Pull the casualty onto their knees.

Now move close to the person, pass your arms under his or her armpits and raise the casualty into a standing position.

3 When the casualty is upright and leaning against you, follow steps 1, 2, 3 and 4 of the first fireman's-lift method described above.

Moving a casualty: two first-aiders

It is easier to move a casualty if two people are available who are able to bear the person's weight. There follow some moving methods that require two first-aiders.

The four-handed seat

Two first-aiders, working and lifting together, can provide a carrier seat for a casualty who cannot walk, but is able to use his or her arms and hands.

1 First, both first-aiders should grip their own left wrists with their own right hands. Using their free left hands, they should then grip the other first-aider's right wrist.

2 Both first-aiders should then squat down to enable the casualty to sit on their gripped hands and pass his or her arms around the neck of each.

3 Both first-aiders should now raise themselves into a standing position.

4 Starting with their outside legs, the first-aiders should then step out at the same time, continuing by walking forwards at an ordinary pace.

1

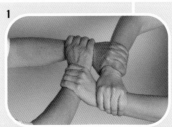

The four–handed seat.

Emergency priorities, actions and techniques

The two-handed seat

The two-handed seat can be used to carry a casualty away from danger when his or her arms have been injured.

1 Having positioned themselves so that they are standing on either side of the casualty and facing each other, the two first-aiders should then squat down.

2 Both first-aiders should now pass the forearm that is nearest to the casualty's body under the casualty's back and then grasp the person's clothing. If there is no clothing to grasp, the first-aiders must grip each other's wrists.

3 Together the first-aiders should raise the casualty's back slightly, before passing their other arms under the middle of the casualty's thighs and then grasping each other's wrists.

4 Both first-aiders should now rise at the same time and start walking in tandem, stepping out with their outside feet first.

2

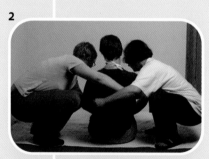

3

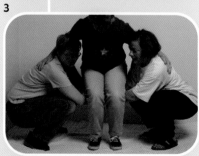

The two-handed seat.

The chair lift

The chair-lift method is suitable when a casualty has to be moved along a corridor and down stairs. The casualty must, however, be conscious, while his or her injuries should not be serious. Make sure that the passage and stairs are free of obstructions and any possible hazards over which the first-aiders could trip. Remember always to inform the casualty when the chair is about to be tilted to avoid causing him or her further distress.

1 Having checked the chair to make sure that it is strong enough to support the casualty's weight, position the casualty so that he or she is sitting well back in it.

2 If possible, secure the casualty's torso and thighs to the chair with scarves or large bandages.

3 With one first-aider standing in front of the chair and the other behind it, and both holding the chair securely, warn the casualty that the chair is about to be tilted before tilting it backwards, about 30° to the horizontal.

4 The first-aider behind the chair should support the chair while the other first-aider, the one facing the casualty, holds the chair by its front legs and moves carefully backwards.

5 If the passageway or staircase is wide enough, the two first-aiders can stand on either side of the chair, each holding one front and one rear leg.

6 Similarly, a disabled casualty can be carried in a wheelchair: having put on the brakes, each first-aider should stand on either side of the chair holding the fixed parts, never the wheels – and take care when gripping armrests and side supports because these may be removable – before moving forward together.

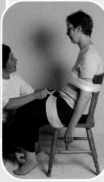

The chair lift.

2

Stretchers

A stretcher is useful when a casualty needs to be removed from imminent danger and carried over some distance. When using a stretcher:

· ensure that the casualty's head, neck and body are aligned and that the airway is not obstructed;

· if possible, drape a blanket across the stretcher before the casualty is placed on it and then wrap the blanket around the person.

Moving a casualty onto a stretcher

When a casualty is unconscious, position the open stretcher against his or her front and then carry the person in the recovery position (see pages 42 to 43). If the casualty is conscious, however, do the following:

1 One first-aider should gently and carefully roll the casualty onto his or her uninjured side, supporting the body behind the shoulders and knees.

2 The other first-aider should then place the open stretcher flat against the casualty's back.

3 With the casualty now lying on it, the stretcher should be gently rolled onto the floor before being lifted up by the first-aiders.

Turning a casualty with a suspected spinal injury

Six people are required to turn a casualty with a suspected spinal injury onto his or her side, which it is vital to do if the person is vomiting to ensure that he or she does not choke. It is also necessary to avoid causing the casualty any distress or discomfort that may cause them to move, potentially injuring themselves further. It is imperative that the casualty's head is always kept in alignment with his or her body.

1 Three people should hold the casualty on one side, two others should hold the casualty's other side, while one further first-aider should hold the casualty's head.

2 With all six helpers working at the same time and speed, the casualty should now be turned carefully, without his or her spine being bent or twisted.

Moving a casualty with a suspected spinal injury

Seven people are needed to move a person with a suspected spinal injury. The first-aider positioned at the casualty's head (a position that provides a view of the axis of the person's body) should be in charge and should instruct the others. Remember that the casualty's head and neck must never move out of alignment with his or her body.

1 With three helpers firmly, but gently, holding the casualty's head, shoulders and pelvis, a fourth helper should place padding made of soft material between the casualty's ankles, knees and thighs.

2 Bind the feet together with a bandage tied in a figure-of-eight pattern to hold the casualty's legs together (see page 83).

3 Three helpers should now be positioned on each side of the casualty, with the remaining first-aider standing at the person's head, carefully holding each side of the head to keep it aligned.

4 With the first-aider at the casualty's head giving instructions, the casualty should now be rolled – with the head, neck and body remaining in alignment – just enough to enable the other first-aiders to slide their arms under casualty's body in preparation for lifting him or her.

Making an improvised stretcher

If none is readily available, it is possible to make an improvised stretcher from sturdy jackets or coats, although this should only be done as a last resort, and tested first by an uninjured person to ensure that they are sufficiently strong.

1 Turn the sleeves of two or three strong jackets or coats inside out.

2 Pass a strong pole through one of the sleeves of each jacket or coat and a second pole through the remaining sleeves.

3 Button or zip up the jackets or coats.

4 Test the makeshift stretcher for strength and stability by asking an uninjured person to lie on it and then lifting up the stretcher to ensure that it can safely bear the person's weight.

5 Move the casualty onto the stretcher using the method described above (see page 30).

Emergency priorities, actions and techniques

Removing helmets and clothing

Most injuries can be inspected and assessed for their severity without having to remove the casualty's clothing: fractures can be felt for, for example, while major wounds will normally be indicated by tears in the casualty's clothing.

There may be times when articles of clothing need to be removed in order to administer the proper treatment, however, but only if it is absolutely essential. When a casualty is conscious, always ask their permission before removing the minimum amount of clothing only, all the while trying to disturb the casualty as little as possible.

Removing helmets

Motorcyclists' helmets should only be removed if absolutely necessary, such as:

· when the casualty's breathing is being obstructed by the helmet;

· when the casualty is not breathing and has no pulse;

· when the casualty is vomiting.

First-aiders are strongly advised not to try to remove a helmet unless it is vital because doing so could cause serious injury, or even death (for instance, if the neck is fractured). In many cases, the motorcyclist's helmet will, however, have prevented the head from being severely injured. When the removal of a helmet is necessary and the casualty is conscious, ask him or her to remove the helmet.

If you need to move a casualty from underneath a motorcycle, be careful not to touch the motorbike's hot engine and exhaust parts. In addition, be sure to note the exact position of the casualty and vehicle before moving them to enable you to report the incident accurately to the emergency services.

Two types of helmet are commonly worn: a protective helmet that covers only the wearer's head, leaving the face exposed (although the helmet may also have a drop-down visor) and a full-face crash helmet that covers both the face and head.

Removing a protective helmet

It is strongly recommended that two first-aiders remove a protective helmet: one should support the casualty's neck and head while the other takes off the helmet.

1 Unfasten or cut the helmet's chin strap.

2 While one first-aider supports the casualty's head and neck, the other should now force the sides of the helmet apart.

3 With the casualty's neck and head still being gently, but firmly, supported by one first-aider, the other first-aider should now lift the helmet upwards, and then backwards, over the casualty's head.

Removing a full-face crash helmet
Two people are again required to effect the safe removal of a full-face helmet: one to support the casualty's head and neck, and the other to remove the helmet.

1 One first-aider should first place his or her hands on each side of the helmet, positioning his or her fingers on the casualty's jaw to keep the head steady. The second first-aider should then cut or loosen the chin strap.

2 The second first-aider – the one who has just cut the strap – should now support the casualty's head by holding it at the base of the skull and jawbone.

3 The first helper should now tilt back the helmet to clear the casualty's chin and nose.

4 The first helper should then tilt the helmet forward to clear the base of the casualty's skull before lifting off the helmet.

Emergency priorities, actions and techniques

Removing a shoe or boot

If a shoe or boot is difficult to remove, it may be necessary to slit the back seam with a sharp blade. Otherwise follow the procedure outlined below.

1 Hold the casualty's ankle firmly, but gently, with one hand.

2 With the other hand, undo – or, if necessary, cut – any shoelace.

3 Still holding the casualty's ankle steady, gently remove the shoe.

1
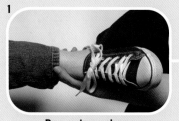

2
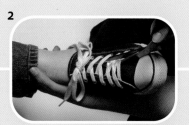

3
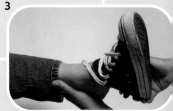

Removing a shoe.

Removing a sock

Only when a sock cannot be slipped off a casualty's foot in the usual way should it be cut with a sharp blade and then removed, as follows.

1 Insert two fingers between the sock and the casualty's leg.

2 Pull the edge of the sock away from the casualty's leg and then cut the sock between your fingers.

1
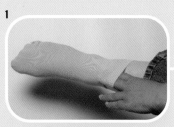

Removing a sock.

Removing trousers

The following tips will ease the removal of a pair of trousers from a casualty:

· when the calf or knee has sustained injury, raise the trouser leg;

· when the injury is to the thigh, pull down the trousers from the waist;

· when the removal of trousers is essential, but proving difficult, carefully slit or cut along the inner seam of the trouser leg to expose the injury.

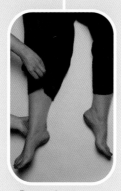

Removing trousers.

Removing jackets, coats or shirts

When the removal of a jacket, coat or shirt is necessary, but proving hard, carefully cutting or slitting the garment along the casualty's injured side may make its removal easier. Otherwise use the following technique.

1 Gently raise the casualty and slip the jacket, coat or shirt over his or her shoulders.

2 Bend the casualty's arm on the uninjured side and then remove the jacket, coat or shirt from this side of the body.

3 Gently pull the jacket, coat or shirt's remaining sleeve off the other arm.

Emergency priorities, actions and techniques

Chapter 2

The signs of life and emergency techniques

The signs of life are breathing and circulation (indicated by the pulse). In an emergency, it is vital that first-aiders ensure that casualties can breathe freely because if the brain is deprived of oxygen at normal temperatures, casualties may suffer serious brain damage, or even die, within a matter of minutes. In addition, without sufficient oxygen, a condition called hypoxia can develop, which can in turn lead to unconsciousness and may sometimes be fatal. Hypoxia can be caused if there is insufficient oxygen in the air, for example, in a smoke-filled room; if there is an obstruction in the airway, perhaps caused by choking; or if the action of the muscles in the chest has been interfered with or paralysed, for instance, when a casualty has been buried or has suffered electrocution. If the casualty cannot breathe unaided, the first-aider must therefore artificially provide him or her with adequate air.

  When faced with a casualty who has collapsed, the first-aider must assess whether the casualty is breathing and has a pulse. Before approaching a casualty, however, first-aiders must always check for danger – to themselves, to others and to the casualty – and should only proceed if it is safe to do so. The next step is to check for a response: is the casualty conscious? To determine this, gently shake the casualty and ask 'Can you hear me?', 'Open your eyes' and 'What is your name?' If there is no response, the casualty is unconscious.

The ABC of resuscitation

There are a number of resuscitation techniques that the first-aider can use, as follows.

A is for airway

When a casualty is unconscious and lying on his or her back, the airway may become blocked by the tongue. Open the airway by lifting the casualty's chin with two fingers and pressing on the forehead to tilt back the head.

Do not leave an unconscious casualty lying face upwards: because the muscles are relaxed, the normal reflexes that ensure an open and clear airway may not be functioning. Indeed, unnecessary deaths are caused by leaving unconscious, but breathing, casualties lying on their backs. Blood or vomit may also enter the air passage because the reflex controlling the opening and closing of the larynx (the 'gagging' action) may not function as it should when foreign matter comes into contact with it. In addition, the inhalation of foreign matter can obstruct the airway and cause a severe form of pneumonia.

The breathing of an unconscious casualty who must be left lying on his or her back rather than in the recovery position (see pages 42 to 43) because there is a risk of spinal injury, must be constantly monitored.

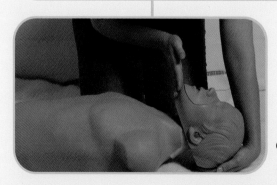

Open the airway by lifting the chin with two fingers and pressing on the forehead to tilt the head back.

B is for breathing

Check for ten seconds to see whether the casualty is breathing. Kneel down beside the casualty, then place your cheek as close as possible to the casualty's mouth and look, listen and feel for signs of breathing:

· look for movement in the chest or abdomen and, if you observe it, check that it is smooth and regular;

· listen for sounds of breathing by placing your ear close to the casualty's mouth and nose;

· feel for the casualty's breath on your cheek. Place your hand on their chest to feel if it is rising (shown below).

If there is no breathing, respiration has stopped and you must supply air to the casualty.

If the chest and abdomen are moving, but there is no air moving in and out of the mouth or nose, the casualty's airway is obstructed and you must therefore clear it. It may be that the casualty's tongue has blocked off the airway, in which case open the airway as described above by tilting the casualty's head.

If the casualty still isn't breathing, there may be an obstruction in the airway that must be cleared immediately.

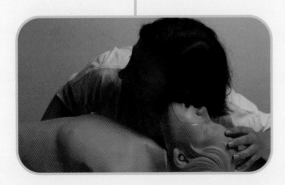

Listen, feel and look for signs of breathing.

The signs of life and emergency techniques

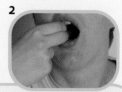

Clearing an obstruction from the airway

Don't waste time! An obstruction must be cleared from the airway immediately, as follows.

1 Turn the casualty's head to one side, keeping the chin to the front and the top of the head to the back.

2 Sweep around the inside of the casualty's mouth with two hooked fingers and remove any foreign matter.

3 Check that the casualty is breathing.

4 Check the casualty's pulse and circulation. (See below).

If the casualty still isn't breathing, start artificial respiration (see pages 42 to 46) immediately.

If the casualty isn't breathing and there is no pulse, start cardiopulmonary resuscitation (CPR, a combination of artificial ventilation and external chest compression immediately, see pages 47 to 53). See also choking, pages 54 to 58.

C is for circulation

The pulse, which indicates the condition of the circulation, is the repeated brief wave of pressure that passes along the arteries every time that the heart's lower chambers contract and squeeze through blood. A pulse rate may vary from slow and full to rapid, weak or fluttering. A weak pulse is a characteristic of shock (see pages 92 to 94) and may be difficult to feel, especially if the first-aider's own heart is beating rapidly in response to the emergency situation, when his or her pulse may be stronger than the casualty's. In such instances, the usual place where one feels for a pulse – on the thumb side of the wrist, 1.5 cm (½ in) above the wrist crease (i.e. up the arm) and 1.5 cm (½ in) away from the edge – may not be reliable and the first-aider should instead feel for the casualty's carotid pulse in the neck. (The carotids are the large arteries that run up each side of the back of the larynx, or Adam's apple.)

Checking the pulse

A first-aider must remain calm when checking a casualty's pulse. If necessary, take a couple of deep breaths to calm yourself and steady your breathing.

1 Place the tips of your index and middle fingers (not your thumb because its strong pulse may be confused with the casualty's) on one side of the casualty's Adam's apple, but without pressing on it.

2 Slide your fingertips firmly, but gently, backwards alongside the Adam's apple so that they pass into the vertical groove between it and the muscle to its side.

3 Feel for the pulse with your fingertips. If you cannot immediately feel a pulse, move your fingertips a little nearer to, and then further from, the Adam's apple. Once you have located the pulse, count the beats per minute and note whether it is strong and regular. An adult heart beats at a rate of 60 to 80 times per minute; a child's up to 100 times per minute.

1

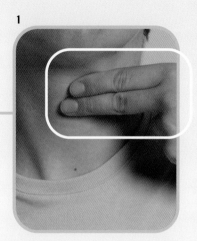

2

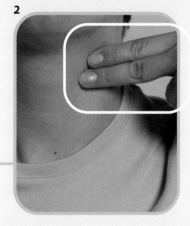

The signs of life and emergency techniques

The recovery position

An unconscious or semiconscious casualty who is breathing should not be left lying on his or her back because the airway is in danger of being blockcd by the tongue in this position. The casualty should instead be moved into the recovery position.

Note that the recovery position should not be used for a casualty who is conscious, or who is likely to regain consciousness, or if there is a risk that the casualty has incurred a spinal injury.

1 Check the casualty's mouth for any obstructions, and clear if necessary.

2 Kneeling down on one side of the casualty, open the airway (see page 38).

3 Straighten the casualty's legs, and then straighten the casualty's arm nearest to you and tuck it, palm facing upwards, under the thigh.

4 Fold the casualty's arm furthest away from you across the casualty's chest, placing the palm of the hand against the cheek nearest to you.

5 Grasp the casualty's thigh furthest from you and pull up the knee, keeping the foot flat on the ground.

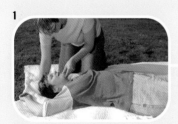

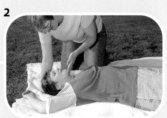

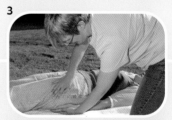

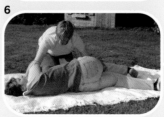

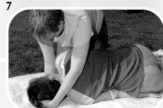

6 With one hand, keep the casualty's palm pressed against his or her cheek to support the head. With your other hand, pull the person's thigh towards you, rolling the casualty onto his or her side as you do so.

7 Gently remove your hand from under the casualty's head and then tilt back the head to keep the airway open.

8 Pull the casualty's uppermost leg up at a right angle to the body to stop it from falling forwards.

9 Remove the casualty's straight arm from under the body to prevent them rolling backwards. Make sure that the airway remains open at all times.

While the casualty is in the recovery position and you're awaiting the arrival of the emergency services, check his or her breathing and circulation at regular intervals. Do not leave the casualty unattended.

For children over one year old who are unconscious, but breathing, use the procedure described above for moving them into the recovery position.

For babies under one year old who are unconscious, but breathing, open the airway and cradle the infant in your arms, the head pointing downwards.

4
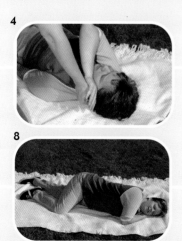

5
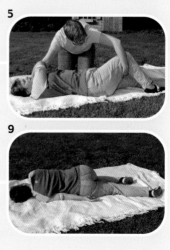

8

9

The signs of life and emergency techniques

The resuscitation of an adult casualty

Artificial respiration (AR), which is also called 'mouth-to-mouth resuscitation' or 'expired-air resuscitation' (EAR), provides an unconscious casualty who is not breathing with an air supply.

The air that we breathe out – the 'expired air' – contains enough oxygen to keep someone else alive, and not only must there be no delay in getting this vital oxygen into the casualty's body, but it must go deep into the lungs. If you cannot see the casualty's chest rise when you blow air into his or her mouth, and then fall when you stop, you are not succeeding and the lungs are not being inflated.

Before approaching a casualty, first-aiders must always:

· check for danger – to themselves, to others and to the casualty – and only proceed if it is safe to do so;

· check for a response: is the casualty conscious? To ascertain this, gently shake the casualty and ask 'Can you hear me?', 'Open your eyes' and 'What is your name?' If there is no response, the casualty is unconscious.

If the casualty has blood, mucus or vomit on his or her face, wipe it away before commencing. If the casualty has bleeding wounds on his or her face or mouth, administer AR through a slit in a clean plastic bag to reduce the risk of cross-infection.

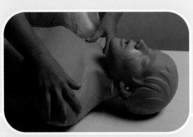

Check for responses by gently shaking the casualty's shoulders and asking 'Can you hear me?'

1

3

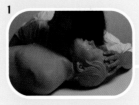

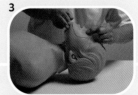

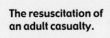

The resuscitation of an adult casualty.

1 Open the airway and then check the casualty's breathing and circulation (pulse): lift the casualty's chin, tilt back the head to keep the airway open and monitor the casualty's breathing for ten seconds.

If the casualty is breathing, turn them into the recovery position (see pages 42 to 43).

2 If the casualty is not breathing, but there is a pulse, remove any visible obstructions from inside his or her mouth using two hooked fingers.

Remember that it is vital that any obstructions are not blown deeper into the casualty's lungs. Keep the airway open by tilting back the head.

3 Pinch the casualty's nostrils closed with one hand. With your other hand, lift the casualty's jaw forwards and upwards, but don't put pressure on the neck.

4 Take a good, deep breath. Open your mouth wide and seal it tightly around the casualty's mouth. Blow strongly into the casualty's mouth to inflate the lungs. At the same time, watch to see if the chest rises.

5 Once the casualty's chest has risen, turn your head to check that the chest then falls.

If the chest does not rise and fall, first check the head-tilt position, then look again for any foreign objects in the airway. Alternatively, you may need to ensure that the nostrils are tightly pinched closed or to blow much harder.

If, after performing these checks, the casualty's chest still does not rise and fall, there must be an airway obstruction beyond the mouth and you will need to follow the procedure for choking (see pages 54 to 58).

6 Administer five full breaths in ten seconds, then check the circulation at the carotid (neck) pulse point for five seconds.

If a pulse is still detectable, continue artificial respiration at a rate of fifteen breaths per minute. Check the casualty's breathing and circulation after one minute, then after every two minutes, until the casualty either begins to breathe again or the emergency services arrive.

4
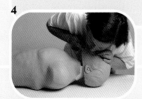

5
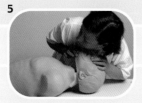

6
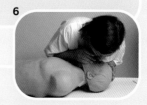

The signs of life and emergency techniques

Mouth-to-nose resuscitation

Mouth-to-nose resuscitation is an alternative method that is used when it is impossible to administer mouth-to-mouth artificial respiration: for example, when a casualty's jaws or teeth – or both – are broken; when the jaws are tightly clenched; when resuscitation is carried out in deep water; or when a child or infant is being resuscitated and your mouth can therefore cover the infant casualty's nose and mouth.

Before proceeding, check for danger and monitor the casualty's response.
1 Kneel down beside the casualty and tilt back his or her head.
2 Close the casualty's mouth and place your thumb on the lower lip to keep the mouth shut. Support the casualty's chin with the remaining fingers of that hand.
3 Take a good, deep breath and open your mouth wide.
4 Seal your mouth around the casualty's nose without squashing the soft part. Breathe strongly into the casualty's nose.
5 After administering one good, strong breath, thereby forcing air into the casualty's lungs and making the chest rise, open the mouth with your thumb to allow the breath to be expelled and check that the chest has fallen.
6 Administer five full breaths in ten seconds, then check the circulation (pulse) at the carotid (neck) pulse point for five seconds.

If a pulse is still detectable, continue artificial respiration at a rate of fifteen breaths per minute. Check the casualty's breathing and circulation after one minute, then after every two minutes, until the casualty either begins to breathe again or the emergency services arrive.

Cardiopulmonary resuscitaion (CPR)

Cardiopulmonary resuscitation (CPR) is a combination of artificial ventilation and external chest compression that is used to resuscitate a casualty who is unconscious, not breathing and has no pulse.

Chest compression was once erroneously called 'external cardiac massage'. In fact, although the heart cannot be massaged from the outside, it can be compressed, which forces the blood to move around the circulation system in the same way as if the heart were functioning (beating) spontaneously.

As long as air is being forced into the lungs at the same time that the chest is being compressed, a casualty who is unconscious, not breathing and has no pulse can be kept alive. And if a casualty is capable of recovery, CPR will often restart the heartbeat, restoring spontaneous breathing.

Before administering CPR, note the following points.

· This technique should only be performed by a trained first-aider or under the guidance of a trained first-aider or the emergency services.

· The casualty's heartbeat must have stopped completely before external chest compression is initiated. A very weak, yet beating, heart can be stopped if this procedure is administered, so never perform CPR on a person whose heart is beating.

· External chest compression without mouth-to-mouth artificial respiration is futile. The casualty must have oxygen, which the first-aider must provide.

The signs of life and emergency techniques

The administration of CPR to an adult casualty by one first-aider

Before administering CPR, check for danger and monitor the casualty's response. Then follow the ABC of resuscitation: clear the airway, check the casualty's breathing and then the circulation (pulse).

If the casualty is not breathing and there is no pulse, inflate the lungs twice using AR (see pages 44 to 46), then check the circulation (pulse) at the carotid (neck) pulse point.

1 If no pulse is detectable, lay the casualty flat and kneel down beside him or her so that one of your knees is level with the chest and the other is level with the head.

2 Locate the lower end of the casualty's breastbone by running your fingers along the lowest rib on each side of the ribcage, moving from the outside inwards.

3 Place your middle finger on the point where the ribs meet and your index finger alongside it. Place the heel of your other hand on the casualty's breastbone, above your two extended fingers – this is the point to which you will apply pressure.

4 Cover your upper hand – the one closest to the casualty's head – with the heel of your other hand, then lock your fingers together.

5 Kneel upright and lean forward so that your shoulders are above the casualty's breastbone. Keep your arms straight and, using the heel of your lower hand only, depress the

1
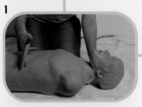

2
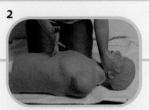

5
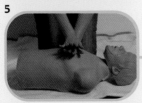

6
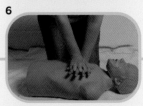

breastbone to a depth of about 4 to 5 cm (11/2 to 2 in) – this is the distance of compression for an adult – without putting pressure on the ribs.

6 Release the pressure without removing your hands and allow the chest to expand. Repeat the compressions, rhythmically depressing and releasing the chest, fifteen times in ten to twelve seconds.

7 Move to the casualty's head and deliver two strong, mouth-to-mouth breaths of air deep into the lungs. Watch carefully to ensure that the casualty's chest rises as the lungs fill with air.

Repeat the cycle of fifteen compressions and two lung inflations, checking the circulation (pulse) after one minute and then after every two minutes.

If there is no pulse, continue CPR.

If there is a pulse, but breathing has not resumed, stop CPR and commence AR, administering ventilations for one minute, then checking the circulation and repeating as necessary.

If both breathing and circulation (pulse) are functioning again, place the casualty in the recovery position, monitor the ABC of resuscitation (airway, breathing and circulation) and wait for the emergency services to arrive.

3
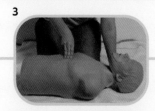

4
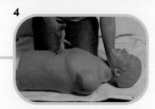

7
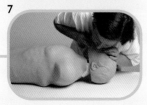

The signs of life and emergency techniques

The administration of CPR to an adult casualty by two first-aiders

Administering CPR is very tiring for one person. Not only can two people administer CPR for longer periods, but also more effectively, especially if they switch over roles at regular intervals.

When two people are available to administer CPR, one person should take charge and supervise the airway, give AR and check the pulse, while the other administers external chest compressions. The first-aider administering external chest compressions should count the compressions out loud so that at the end of the fifth compression AR is administered without a pause. Timing is vital: do not attempt to inflate the casualty's lungs while the chest is being compressed.

Before administering CPR, check for danger and monitor the casualty's response. Then follow the ABC of resuscitation: clear the airway, check the casualty's breathing and then the circulation (pulse).

1 The first first-aider should start with two inflations, then check again for a pulse.

2 If no pulse is detectable, the second first-aider should now administer five chest compressions, after which the first first-aider should administer one inflation in five seconds. The neck pulse should be checked every two minutes.

3 Repeat the compressions and inflation until the casualty begins to recover and the emergency services arrive.

If there is no pulse, continue CPR.

If there is a pulse, but breathing has not resumed, stop CPR and commence AR, administering ventilations for one minute, then checking the circulation and repeating as necessary.

If both breathing and circulation (pulse) are functioning again, place the casualty in the recovery position, monitor the ABC of resuscitation (airway, breathing and circulation) and wait for the emergency services to arrive.

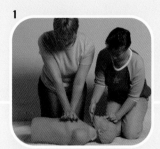
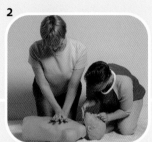
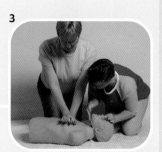

Resuscitation techniques: infant and child casualties

The resuscitation techniques described above for adult casualties are suitable for children over eight years old. For younger children, and babies under one year old, the resuscitation techniques and procedures are slightly different, however. When administering AR to a baby, you will need to seal your mouth completely over the baby's nose and mouth and use quick, shallow puffs of air because too much pressure may distend the baby's stomach. For older children, gently pinch their nostrils and cover their mouth with yours, as you would when treating an adult casualty.

In all cases, start by checking for a response by very gently shaking a baby's or young child's shoulders and calling his or her name. (Even very young babies have been known to respond to the sound of a familiar voice saying their name.) If you don't know the baby's or child's name, a term of endearment may also provoke a response. If there is no response, the baby or child is unconscious and you should then follow the ABC of resuscitation: clear the airway, check the casualty's breathing and then the circulation (pulse).

The signs of life and emergency techniques

1a

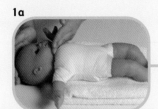

1b

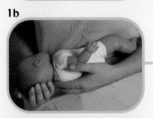

2

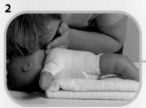

3

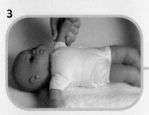

4

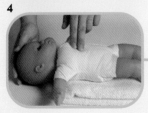

Infant casualties

Resuscitate an unconscious baby as follows. For very small babies, you will need to lie them on a towel or pad so that they lie flat – as babies heads are so large, if you lie them flat on a hard, level surface, their airway will be obstructed.

1a Open the airway by placing one finger gently under the chin and then lifting it to open the airway without pressing on the soft tissue under the chin. Place your cheek close to the baby's face to feel, listen and look for the signs of breathing.

1b If the infant is breathing, put it in the recovery position by cradling the baby in your arms with its head tilting downwards.

2 If the baby is not breathing, check for, and if you find any, remove obstructions in the child's mouth. Gently lift the chin, cover the baby's mouth and nose with your mouth and then puff gently, using just enough pressure to inflate the baby's chest. Administer five puffs of air.

3 Check the circulation (pulse) by applying two fingers to the brachial pulse point on the inside of the baby's upper arm and holding them there for ten seconds.

If a pulse is detectable, continue to administer AR.

4 If the baby's pulse is not detectable, or is less than 60, start CPR by placing two fingers on the baby's lower breastbone and pressing down to a depth of 1.5 cm (½ in).

If you are a lone first-aider, apply fifteen compressions, followed by two quick puffs of air within ten seconds.

If you have assistance, apply five compressions, followed by one quick puff of breath within three seconds.

Child casualties (under eight years old)

Resuscitate an unconscious child under the age of eight as follows.

1 Place two fingers under the child's chin and gently lift it to open the airway. Place your cheek close to the child's face to feel, look and listen for the signs of breathing.

If the child is breathing, place it in the recovery position.

2 If the child is not breathing, gently pinch the nostrils closed and then seal your mouth over his or her mouth. Apply five quick, shallow breaths and then check the circulation (pulse) at the carotid pulse point for ten seconds.

If a pulse is detectable, continue to administer AR until the child either recovers or the emergency services arrive, checking the circulation (pulse) every minute.

3 If no pulse is detectable, administer CPR. Locate the middle of the child's breastbone and place the heel of your hand slightly below this point. Your fingers should be relaxed, slightly raised and pointing across the child's chest.

4 Using the heel of this hand alone, depress the child's chest to a depth of about 2 to 3 cm (¾ to 1 in), working gently and rhythmically.

If you are a lone first-aider, apply fifteen compressions, followed by two quick, shallow breaths within ten seconds.

If you have assistance, apply five compressions, followed by one quick, shallow breath within three seconds.

The signs of life and emergency techniques

Choking

Choking on an object or piece of food can happen to anyone at any age. Choking can be caused by laughing or crying while eating; running and stumbling while eating; not chewing food properly; swallowing a bone or splinters of a bone; or inhaling while eating or drinking.

If an object or piece of food becomes stuck in someone's throat and blocks off the airway, the person may start coughing, may clutch or point to his or her throat, may have difficulty speaking and may become distressed. An adult casualty's face may become very red, while a child or baby's face may become flushed. If the blockage remains stuck, the casualty may lose consciousness. Prompt first aid is vital in all cases.

The first step is to encourage the casualty to cough up the obstruction. If this fails to dislodge it, 'bending and slapping' should be tried, a technique that can be performed on both adults and children (don't be afraid of hurting a child by administering sharp slaps because this is an emergency and his or her life is in danger).

If 'bending and slapping' fails – and only then, because it may cause internal injuries – the abdominal-thrust method should be used. Abdominal thrusts require considerable force to compress the upper abdomen and push upwards on the diaphragm, the muscle that forms the floor of the chest. This should cause a sudden rise in pressure within the lungs, which should drive out the obstruction – a bit like a cork exiting a champagne bottle. Do not be afraid to administer abdominal thrusts if all of the other methods have failed because if there is a complete obstruction of the airway, the casualty may die unless it is removed.

If the casualty is a baby, infant or child, or any casualty who has lost consciousness at any time, hospital treatment is vital because the airway may have been injured or have become swollen. Hospital treatment is also necessary if the casualty continues to experience residual breathing difficulties after the obstruction has been removed.

Treating a choking adult

The first-aider's primary aim is to clear the obstruction from the casualty's throat.

1 Tell the casualty to bend forward at the waist. Stand behind the casualty and administer five sharp slaps with the flat of your hand to the casualty's back, between the shoulder blades. Then check the casualty's mouth to see if the object has been dislodged.

2 If the back slaps have failed to dislodge the obstruction, you will have to administer abdominal thrusts. Stand behind the casualty, pass your arms around him or her and place a clenched fist – with your thumb tucked in over the upper abdomen – just below the ribs.

3 Grasp your clenched fist with your other hand and then pull inwards and upwards up to five times. Check the casualty's mouth to see if the object has been dislodged.

4 If this fails to dislodge the object, call for an ambulance and repeat steps 1 to 3 until emergency services arrive.

1
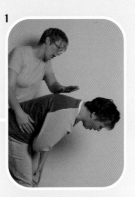

2
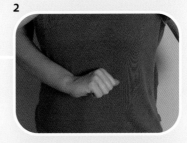

3
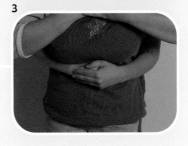

The signs of life and emergency techniques

If an adult casualty loses consciousness

If the casualty becomes unconscious, follow the procedure outlined below.

1 Turn the casualty onto his or her side, tilt back the head and administer five sharp slaps with the flat of your hand to the casualty's back, between the shoulder blades. Then check the casualty's mouth with your fingers to see if the obstruction has come loose.

2 If this fails to dislodge the obstruction, you will have to administer abdominal thrusts. Turn the casualty onto his or her back, tilt the chin upwards and gently push back the head.

3 Kneel astride, or, failing that, alongside, the casualty's upper thighs, facing the head. Place the heel of one hand on the centre of the casualty's upper abdomen, between the navel and the angle joined by the ribs, and then cover it with your other hand. Now forcibly thrust inwards and upwards up to five times.

4 Check to see if the object has been dislodged by sweeping two hooked fingers inside the casualty's mouth. If it has, remove the object, check the casualty's breathing and circulation (pulse) and administer resuscitation if necessary.

Treating a choking child
(aged between one and seven years old)

The following technique should be used to treat a choking child.

1 Stand or kneel behind the child, tell him or her to lean forwards and then administer five sharp slaps with the flat of your hand to the child's back, between the shoulder blades. Don't be afraid of hurting the child – this is an emergency! Then sweep two hooked fingers inside and around the child's mouth to clear any obstruction.

2 If this fails, administer five chest thrusts. Stand or kneel behind the child, hold one fist against the breastbone, grasp your fist with your other hand and press inwards. Check the mouth and clear any obstruction.

3 If this fails, repeat the back slaps described in step 1 and check the mouth once more.

4 If the obstruction remains in place, apply five abdominal thrusts. Stand or kneel behind the child, hold a clenched fist against the abdomen, grasp your fist with your other hand and then press sharply inwards. Now check the child's mouth again.

5 If this fails, repeat step 1, then step 2, then step 3 until the emergency services arrive.

The signs of life and emergency techniques

Treating a choking baby (up to one year old)

Although it is vital to remove an obstruction from a baby's or infant's throat when he or she begins to choke, do not put your fingers down the throat to feel for, or attempt to remove, the obstruction. Do not use abdominal thrusts on a baby or infant either. Instead, follow the procedure outlined below.

1 Lay the baby or infant face down along one of your forearms and then administer five sharp slaps to the back with the flat of your hand. Do not be afraid of hurting the baby – this is an emergency, and you must act quickly and confidently.

2 Sweep one finger in and around the inside of the baby's mouth to see the obstruction has been dislodged; if it has, remove it.

3 Lay the baby or infant face up on your arm. Using two fingers only, apply up to five downward thrusts to the chest before checking the baby's mouth again.

4 If the obstruction has still not been dislodged, repeat steps 1 to 3 three times and then call the emergency services, keeping the baby or infant with you all of the time. Continue to repeat steps 1, 2 and 3 until help arrives.

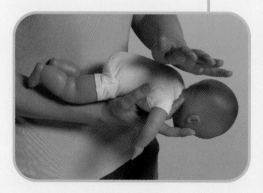

The signs of recovery

When a casualty begins to show signs of recovery, the first-aider needs to check his or her ABC – airway, breathing and circulation (pulse) – to place the casualty in the recovery position, if possible, and then to continue to monitor the ABC until help arrives. In addition, be ready to administer further resuscitation if necessary.

The first-aider must always look, listen and feel for the signs of recovery:

· look at the casualty's skin tone: any blue-, grey- or purple-coloured tones should disappear as the skin regains a healthy colour;

· listen for the sound of the casualty groaning, coughing or spluttering as spontaneous breathing recommences;

· feel for the pulse returning, as well as movement and resistance as you administer AR and spontaneous breathing recommences.

Only when a casualty has resumed spontaneous breathing can the first-aider treat such serious, life-threatening injuries as shock, major bleeding or burns.

Remember, too, that if the casualty is conscious, you should constantly reassure him or her, and that when the emergency services arrive, you should tell them what type of treatment you have administered.

Chapter 3

Dressings, bandages and slings

A properly equipped first-aid kit can save vital minutes – and lives – in an emergency because everything that you need will be conveniently found in one place. Even when a minor injury like a cut finger occurs, we all too often end up running around like headless chickens looking for a clean piece of cloth for a bandage, a pair of scissors to cut it with or simply an adhesive plaster dressing. Every home should house a clearly labelled first-aid kit, and you should also ideally carry one in your car, trailer or boat and in your suitcase when you go on holiday.

You can buy first-aid kits in various sizes from supermarkets, pharmacists, DIY and motor-parts stores, but you could also construct your own and keep it in a plastic sandwich box with a securely fitting, water- and air-tight lid. First-aid kits should always be stored in a childproof container and kept in an easily accessible place that is out of children's reach.

Keep your copy of The First-aid Handbook with your kit so that you can refer to it quickly. It's also a good idea to stick a card to the kit listing the phone numbers of your doctor and local pharmacist and detailing any allergies, medical problems or prescribed medications for each member of the family. Check your first-aid kit regularly and replace any items as you use them up, along with those that are missing, worn, damaged or dirty or have passed their use-by date.

Putting together a first-aid kit

The items listed below should form the basis of your first-aid kit, but remember that you can add to them. If you have young children, you may want to include a thermometer, for example, or if you are a keen hiker or camper, such items as blankets and plastic or foil survival bags. These survival bags are also recommended for motorists, who should carry a red, reflective warning triangle, too, either to place near a road accident or simply to warn other motorists of a mechanical breakdown.

First-aid kits for use in cars should be stored in waterproof containers that should also be soft to prevent them from injuring passengers in the event of an accident. If you are motoring abroad, check the requirements of the countries in which you will be driving: some countries insist that every car contains a first-aid kit, while others may also require you to carry additional emergency equipment, such as a fire extinguisher. Before setting off on your trip, check with your own motoring organisation, which will give you the necessary advice.

Most prepackaged first-aid kits also include such items as plastic disposable gloves, while some even contain a plastic face shield through which artificial respiration (AR) can be administered without making direct contact with a casualty's mouth. Both items guard against cross-infection (see pages 15 to 17) and are vital when attending an emergency as a first-aider.

First-aid kit essentials

The following are essential components of any first-aid kit:
· dressings: assorted sterile gauze, field and adhesive dressings;
· bandages: roller (and conforming) and triangular;
· sterile swabs;
· scissors: round-ended and used exclusively for first aid;
· safety pins (in a variety of sizes) and adhesive fabric tape.

Dressings, bandages and slings

Dressings

Dressings are used to control bleeding, help blood to clot, protect wounds, absorb any fluid from wounds, minimise swelling, prevent infection and ease pain. Although dressings should be non-adhesive and sterile, a single square of clean, dry, absorbent non-fluffy cloth can be used in an emergency.

Gauze dressings are non-adhesive layers of gauze wrapped in sterile covers. They are used for large wounds that need a light covering, such as a burn, and can be secured with adhesive strapping or fabric tape if bandages are either unavailable or difficult to apply.

It would be sensible to include two large, two medium-sized and two small sterile field dressings in your first-aid kit. Designed for easy application and convenient to use, these consist of layers of gauze and a cotton-wool padding already attached to a roller bandage and packaged in a sterile wrapping. They are the best first-aid dressings for large wounds, but are available in a range of shapes and sizes.

Assorted adhesive dressings, or plasters, are sold in a wide range of shapes, sizes and colours, including 'fun' versions for children. Clear, waterproof and elasticated-fabric plasters are all available, as well as the blue plasters used by professional kitchen and catering staff and ones specially designed for fingers and heels. Plasters will not stick to the skin around a wound unless it is clean and dry.

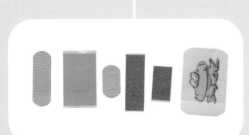

Assorted adhesive dressings, available in a range of sizes.

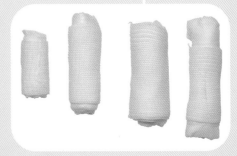

Rolled field dressings: layers of gauze and cotton-wool dressing attached to a roller bandage.

Bandages

Bandages are used to maintain direct pressure to control bleeding, to keep dressings in place, to prevent the undesirable movement of an injured limb, to support an injured limb or joint and to prevent swelling. In some instances, bandages are also used to help to lift and carry casualties. There are two main types of bandage: roller (and conforming) and triangular.

Roller bandages are made of cotton, gauze or linen, are available in rolls of up to 5 metres (5 yards) and come in varying widths to suit different parts of the body: 2.5 centimetres (1 inch) for fingers; 5 centimetres (2 inches) for hands; 5 or 6 centimetres (2 or 2½ inches) for arms; 7.5 or 9 centimetres (3 or 3½ inches) for legs; and 10 or 15 centimetres (4 or 6 inches) for torsos. A ready-made first-aid kit will contain a selection of roller bandages, but you can also make your own from clean, dry strips of cotton fabric, cut to the desired width and length and then rolled up tightly.

Elasticated crêpe bandages, called conforming bandages, are easy to apply, and because they 'conform' to the body's contours, maintain an even pressure over a wound or injury.

Triangular bandages are used as slings for support and protection, for securing dressings to the head, hand or foot and, by folding them, to make broad and narrow bandages for immobilising fractures and securing dressings to wrists and ankles (see pages 83 to 85). Although you can buy ready-made triangular bandages, it is simple – and cheaper – to make your own by cutting a piece of fabric (cotton sheeting, linen or calico are best) measuring not less than 1 metre square (1 yard square) diagonally in half.

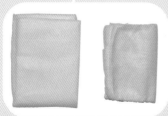

Large and small triangular bandages are used for slings and securing dressings.

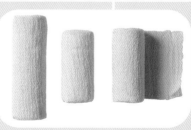

Elasticated crepe conforming bandages mould to the body's contours.

Dressings, bandages and slings

Sterile swabs

As long as the wound is not too large and any bleeding has been controlled, sterile swabs or some clean, dry squares of cotton and a bottle of antiseptic solution formulated for cleaning cuts and grazes can be used to clean both the wound and the surrounding skin.

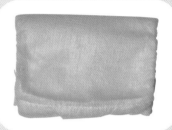

Sterile swabs.

Safety pins.

Scissors

Tearing up a piece of fabric with which to make a bandage or sling looks easy in the movies; it's much more difficult in real life, however, so make sure that your first-aid kit contains a pair of scissors. These should be round-ended – so that you don't end up stabbing an already distressed casualty – and should only be used for first-aid purposes.

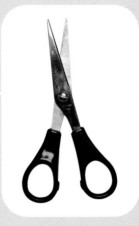

Scissors.

Safety pins and adhesive fabric tape

Bandages can be secured in a number of ways:
· with a safety pins;
· with adhesive fabric strapping or tape (which come in rolls of different widths and lengths) or, in an emergency, even adhesive office tape;
· by cutting the end of a bandage in half along its length, wrapping the two ends in opposite directions around the injured limb and then tying a reef knot (see page 73);
· with the special clips that are already attached to some ready-made bandages.

Whichever method you end up using, it's advisable to equip your first-aid kit with some safety pins and adhesive fabric tape.

Useful additions to your first-aid kit

As well as the essential items listed above, it's a good idea to include in your first-aid kit some, or all, of the following further useful items:
· a pair of flat-ended tweezers, without serrated edges, for removing splinters;
· hydrocortisone cream with which to treat bites and stings and to relieve sunburn;
· anti-diarrhoea preparations;
· temperature-lowering medication, such as aspirin or paracetamol tablets, or those formulated especially for children, with which to treat fevers, as well as headaches and menstrual cramps;
· calamine lotion, an anti-inflammatory lotion that soothes sunburn and rashes;
· clove oil, an essential oil that can be rubbed on the gums and teeth to relieve pain and inflammation until you can get to a dentist.

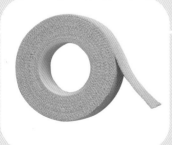

Fabric tape.

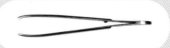

Tweezers.

Dressings, bandages and slings

Applying dressings, bandages and slings

There are a number of different ways of applying various dressings and bandages, depending on the injury. Again, although you can buy dressings and bandages, you may have to improvise in an emergency and use towels or linen – perhaps even a clean handkerchief – to help to save a life.

Remember that a dressing should always be large enough to cover the wound and should extend at least 2.5 centimetres (1 inch) all around it. A dressing should ideally be sterile, to prevent the wound from becoming infected, and should be made of a material that allows sweat to evaporate (if the dressing becomes saturated with accumulated sweat, bacteria may grow and infect the wound).

Applying a dressing: the rules

There are a few rules to remember when applying a dressing.

· Do not place fluffy materials, such as cotton wool, directly on a wound because the fibres will stick to it.

· Do not touch a wound or any part of a dressing that will come into contact with it.

· Whenever possible, wash your hands thoroughly before handling a sterile dressing.

· Both the wound and the surrounding skin must be cleaned thoroughly before applying a dressing, but only if the wound is not too large and the bleeding has been controlled.

· To absorb fluid and control bleeding, secure some cotton-wool padding over a field dressing with a bandage.

· To ward off infection, replace a dressing that has slipped from a wound, to an area of the skin that has not been cleaned, with a fresh dressing.

· Do not slide a dressing onto a wound from an area of skin that has not been cleaned; instead position, and then place, the dressing directly over the wound.

· Do not talk, cough or sneeze over a wound or dressing.

Applying an adhesive dressing

Before applying a plaster or adhesive dressing, wash your hands thoroughly and check that the casualty is not allergic to the adhesive dressing (if so, use a sterile dressing instead). Clean the wound and surrounding skin, and allow it to dry, to ensure that the adhesive sticks to the skin.

1 Unwrap the adhesive dressing and hold it with the central pad facing downwards.

2 Taking care not to touch the central pad, gently peel back the protective plastic strip until the gauze pad is exposed, but don't pull it off completely.

3 Place the central pad over the wound, pull away the protective strip and press the edges of the adhesive dressing firmly against the casualty's skin.

Do not leave an adhesive dressing in place for more than twenty-four hours.

1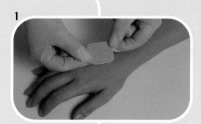

2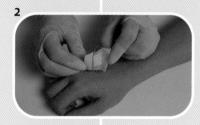

3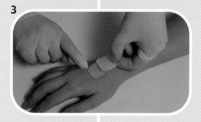

Dressings, bandages and slings

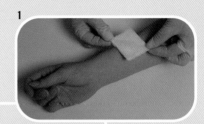

Applying a gauze dressing

Before applying a gauze dressing, wash your hands thoroughly. Remove the gauze dressing from its protective wrapper, holding it by the edges only to keep it as sterile as possible.

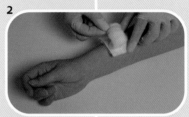

1 Holding the gauze dressing by the edges, carefully position it directly over the wound and then press it down so that it covers the wound. Don't slide the dressing into place.

2 Cover the gauze dressing with a cotton-wool pad.

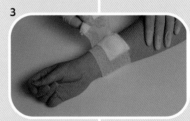

3 Fix the gauze dressing and cotton-wool pad in place with a bandage or adhesive fabric tape.

  If the wound continues to bleed, do not remove the gauze dressing because this will impair any clot that is beginning to form and may make the bleeding worse. Instead, position another large gauze dressing over the top and then bandage it firmly in place. (For more on severe bleeding, see pages 97 to 102.)

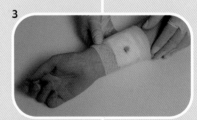

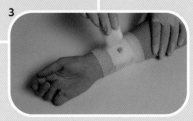

Applying a sterile field dressing

Wash your hands thoroughly before removing the field dressing's inner and outer wrappings. Then support the injured limb in the desired position.

1 With the rolled part uppermost, unroll the short end of the bandage until the end of the sterile dressing is visible.

2 Hold the bandage so that the dressing is over the wound, with the gauze side above it. Now place the dressing on the wound.

3 Holding the dressing's pad in place over the wound, wrap the short end of the bandage over the pad and affected limb (do this only once).

4 Securely bind the affected limb with the long end of the bandage, starting below the site of the injury and working up the limb. The bandage should cover all of the sterile dressing.

5 Tie the two ends of the bandage together using a reef knot (see page 73).

1
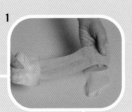

2
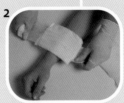

3
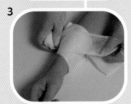

4
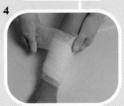

4
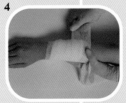

5
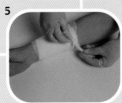

Dressings, bandages and slings

Applying a bandage: the rules

Observing the following tips will make bandaging a casualty easier.

· Make sure that the bandage is rolled up tightly.

· Ensure that when you hold the bandage, the rolled-up part is uppermost.

· Support the part of the body to which you will be applying the bandage.

· Apply the bandage while the casualty is sitting or lying down.

· Sit or stand in front of the casualty and work from the injured side.

· When the casualty is lying down, pass bandages under the natural hollows of the body – the ankles, knees, back and neck – and then ease them into position.

· Because the tissues around an injury may swell, check bandages frequently to ensure that they are not becoming too tight. Although bandages should be wound firmly enough to control bleeding, keep the dressing in position or prevent movement of the injured limb, they should not be so tight that they interfere with the circulation.

· When bandaging a hand or foot, leave the finger- or toenails exposed so that you can check that the bandage is not cutting off the circulation (see page 73).

· Begin bandaging below the site of the injury and work up the limb so that you are bandaging from joint to joint: from ankle to knee or from wrist to elbow.

· When bandages are used to immobilise a fracture, ensure that there is plenty of padding between the limb or any bony areas, such as the knees and ankles, and the bandage.

· When bandaging to immobilise a fracture, tie a reef knot (see page 73) at the uninjured side of the body or limb.

· When bandaging to maintain direct pressure and to control bleeding, tie a reef knot (see page 73) over the pad or dressing.

· Always apply a bandage with care because moving any part of the casualty unnecessarily may cause pain and shock (see pages 92 to 94), and be especially careful to avoid moving the limb when bandaging a fracture.

Tying a reef knot

A reef knot is often used to secure bandages (and slings) because, although it does not come undone by itself, it is easy to untie. Because it's a flat knot, it won't protrude into a wound and cause further discomfort either. 'Left over right and under, right over left and under' is a simple way of remembering how to tie a reef knot.
1 Holding both ends of the bandage, place the left-hand end over the right-hand end.

2 Take what is now the right-hand end under, and then back up over, the left-hand end.
3 Bring the two ends together and then place the right-hand end over the left-hand end.
4 Take the right-hand end under, and then back up over, the left-hand end.
5 Pull on the two ends to tighten and secure the knot.

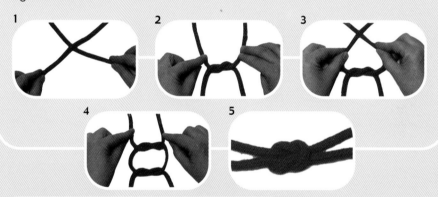

Finger- or toenail test for circulation

Press a finger- or toenail of an injured limb until it turns white. When the pressure is released, it should turn pink again. If the circulation is affected, however, the finger- or toenail will remain white or blue and the extremities will feel cold.

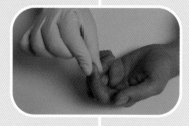

Dressings, bandages and slings

Applying roller or conforming bandages

There are various ways in which roller or conforming bandages can be applied, depending on the site of the injury.

Spiral bandaging

Support the injured part of the casualty, in the position in which it is to be bandaged, with your hand. Hold the bandage with the rolled-up part facing upwards.

1 Place the tail of the bandage on the limb and make a firm, slightly slanted, turn to secure it. Begin bandaging from below the site of the injury up the limb, and from the inside to the outside, unrolling only a few inches of the bandage at a time.

2 As you work up the limb, continue making slanted turns, spiralling the bandage around the limb. Each turn should cover two-thirds of the previous turn.

3 Finish bandaging with a horizontal turn above the injured site and then fold in the edge of the bandage, either on the outside of the limb or well away from the injury, to secure it. Now check the casualty's circulation.

Bandaging knees or elbows

With the casualty either lying or sitting down, ask him or her to support the injured limb in the position that is the most comfortable. Remember to keep the rolled-up part of the bandage uppermost and to unwind only a few inches at a time.

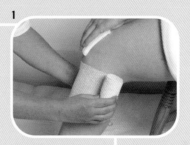

1 Hold the tail of the bandage against one side of the kneecap or elbow. Make one straight turn, taking the rolled 'head' of the bandage over the kneecap or elbow and around the joint.

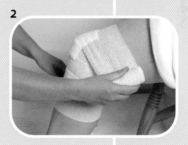

2 Wind the bandage around the upper leg or arm, covering the top edge of the first turn.

3 Wind the bandage around the lower leg or arm, covering the lower edge of the first turn.

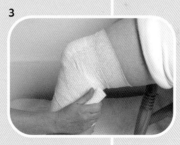

4 Continue to wind the bandage around the upper leg or arm, then the lower leg or arm, but don't cover more than two-thirds of each previous turn.

5 Complete your bandaging by winding one or two slightly slanting turns around the upper leg or arm and then securing the bandage on the outside of the leg or arm. Check the casualty's circulation using the finger- or toenail test (see page 73).

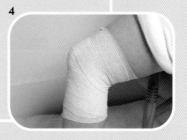

Dressings, bandages and slings

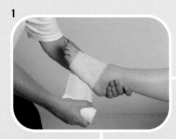

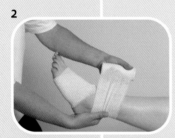

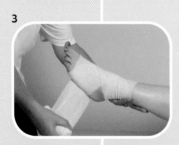

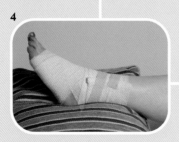

Bandaging feet and ankles
With the casualty either sitting or lying down, raise and support the injured foot to keep it immobilised.

1 Anchor the tail of the bandage under the foot and then wrap the bandage around the instep (do this only once).

2 Pass the bandage diagonally across the top of the foot in a figure-of-eight pattern, then make a straight turn around the ankle and underneath the instep.

3 Continue to bandage in figure-of-eight turns around the foot and ankle, making sure that each turn overlaps the previous one so that the instep and heel are covered and the ankle is supported.

4 Finish off by making a straight turn around the ankle and then secure the bandage's folded edge on the outside of the ankle. Check the circulation using the toenail test (see page 73).

Bandaging wrists

Ask the casualty to raise and support the injured limb to keep it immobilised.

1 Anchor the tail of the bandage to the casualty's wrist by making a horizontal turn around the wrist with the 'head' of the bandage.

2 Take the bandage diagonally across the palm of the hand so that it passes between the thumb and the fingers.

3 Take the bandage around the back of the hand, then diagonally across the palm, then down to, and around, the back of the wrist.

4 Continue to wind the bandage across the palm (as in step 2), around the back of the hand, up around the palm and then around the back of the wrist (as in step 3) until the wrist is adequately supported. Secure the end of the bandage.

5 Check the casualty's circulation using the fingernail test (see page 73).

1
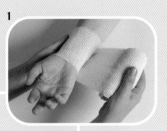

2
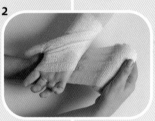

3
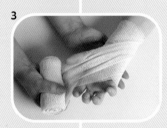

4
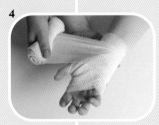

5
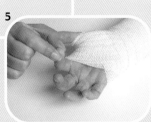

Dressings, bandages and slings

Bandaging the palm of the hand
Because several blood vessels may be damaged, a wound to the palm of the hand can cause severe bleeding that is often difficult to control. If the wound has an object embedded in it, treat it as described on page 80. If the wound contains no foreign matter, treat it as described below.
1 Check the wound to make sure that there are no objects embedded in it.

Ask the casualty to raise and support the arm above chest level. Place a sterile dressing on the wound and ask the casualty to clench his or her fist over the pad.
2 With the casualty's fist still clenched, place the tail of the bandage along the wrist and the 'head' of the bandage over the top of the fist.

1

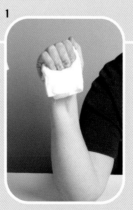

2

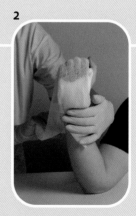

3 Bring the 'head' of the bandage around the fist, under the thumb – leaving the thumb free and uncovered – and then around the fist once more.

4 Take the 'head' end of the bandage over the top of the clenched fist and tie it to the tail end with a reef knot.

5 Check the casualty's circulation, both by taking the pulse at the wrist (see page 40) and by lightly pinching the thumbnail (see page 73).

6 Support the casualty's arm, if possible by using an elevation sling (see page 88), and then seek medical attention.

3

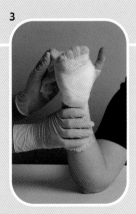

4

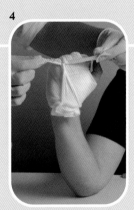

5

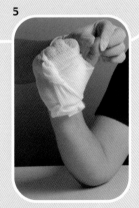

Dressings, bandages and slings

Bandaging wounds with objects embedded in them
If dirt or loose particles of foreign material are embedded in minor wounds, these should be washed out. Larger foreign bodies – shards of glass, metal or wood, for example – which have penetrated the tissue, should not be removed, however.
· Never try to remove foreign bodies from deep wounds because this may precipitate severe bleeding or cause profound physiological damage.
· Do not put pressure on the embedded object.
· Do not try to shorten the embedded object.
· If an object is large, embedded in a lower limb, near a vital organ or the eyes, call an ambulance.

You can, however, bandage the wound before seeking medical attention. First ask the casualty to lie down and then, if possible, raise and support the injured part.
1 Control any bleeding by pinching the edges of the wound together around the embedded object. Do not put any pressure on the object.
2 Cover the wound and the protruding object with sterile gauze, if it is available, or a piece of clean material, such as a handkerchief.

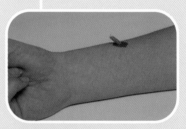

1

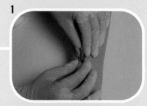

2

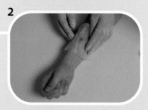

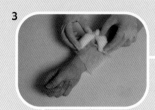

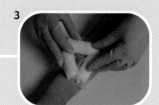

3 Very carefully place some padding on top of the gauze. (Do not press the gauze tightly onto the object in case you drive it further into the wound.) Because the padding must be higher than the protruding object, use rolled-up 'sausages' of cotton wool or a ring pad (see page 82).

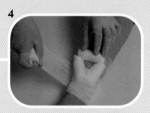

4 Place the tail of the bandage over part of the padding nearest to you and then make two horizontal turns around the casualty's limb with the 'head' of the bandage to secure it.

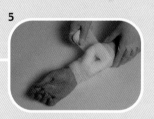

5 Pass the 'head' of the bandage around the limb on either side of the padding.

6 Continue to wind the bandage around the limb, making diagonal turns above and below the injury on either side of the padding, until the dressing is secure and firm. Keep the injured limb raised, supported and as still as possible before seeking medical attention.

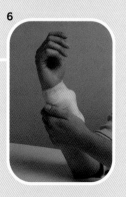

Dressings, bandages and slings

Making a ring pad

In some instances, such as when an object is embedded in a wound, or when a broken bone is protruding through a casualty's skin (see open fractures, page 137), although it is vital to control bleeding, to protect the wound from infection and to immobilise the affected area, direct pressure must not be placed on the embedded object or bone in case further injury is caused. The area around the injury consequently needs to be padded to hold the bandage away from the wound, object or bone, and a good way of doing this is to make a ring pad.

1 Wind one end of a narrow bandage around your fingers to make a loop.

2 Bring the other end through the loop and wrap it over, and under, the loop until you have produced a firm ring.

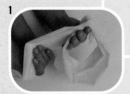
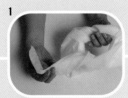
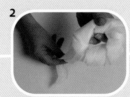
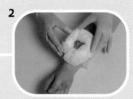

Using Gauze pads

Pads can be tricky to keep in place, and ring pads can be fiddly to make, so if you have a ready supply of gauze pads, you may find it easier to use these to treat an embedded object.

1 First fold a gauze square into quarters, and cut off one corner.

2 This leaves you with a square with a hole roughly in the middle.

3 Continue cutting gauze pads, and place them over the embedded object until it is well padded. This is an easy, effective method to protect such a wound.

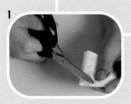
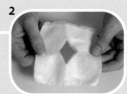
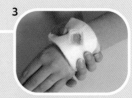

Applying triangular bandages

Triangular bandages are used as slings for support and protection, as well as for securing dressings to heads, feet or hands when pressure does not need to be applied to control bleeding, as in the case of a burn.

Triangular bandages can also be folded to make broad or narrow bandages with which to secure dressings to wrist and ankle joints when no other type of bandage is available, and to tie a figure-of-eight bandage around the feet and ankles when immobilising a fracture or when moving a casualty with a suspected spinal injury away from further danger.

Folding triangular bandages into broad or narrow bandages

Make a broad or narrow bandage from a triangular bandage as follows.
1 Open a triangular bandage and lay it on a flat surface.
2 Fold the point of the bandage over so that it meets the base of the triangle.

3 Fold the bandage in half again to make a broad bandage.
4 To make a narrow bandage, simply fold a broad bandage in half once more along its length.

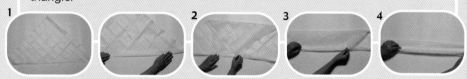

1   2   3   4

Applying a figure-of-eight bandage

You will need to start with a ready-made broad bandage.
1 Pass one end of the broad bandage under the natural hollows of the casualty's ankles and then pull the bandage through until both ends are of equal length on either side of the ankles.

2 Bring the two ends of the bandage upwards and then cross them above the ankles.
3 Take the two ends downwards, around the outside edges of the feet, and then secure the bandage under the soles with a reef knot (see page 73).

Dressings, bandages and slings

Applying a triangular bandage to a foot or hand

Apply a triangular bandage to an injured foot or hand as follows.

1 Place the casualty's foot or hand on the triangular bandage so that the point is pointing away from the toes or fingers. Make sure that there is enough width in the long edge of bandage so that when it is folded upwards it covers the heel and ankle or the heel of the hand.

2 Bring the point of the bandage up to rest on the lower shin or lower forearm.

3 Bring the ends of the bandage over the front of the foot or hand and cross them over each other.

4 Take the ends behind the ankle or wrist, cross them over and then bring them round to the front again.

5 Using a reef knot (see page 73), tie the two ends where the bandage lies over the foot and ankle or hand and wrist.

6 Lift the point of the bandage over the reef knot and secure it to the bandage over the instep (or back of the wrist if bandaging a hand) either with a safety pin or by tucking the end up, and under, the knot.

Where pressure is needed to control bleeding from the palm of the hand, place a pad (or else a tightly folded clean handkerchief, a roll of bandage or a clean cloth wrapped around a smooth pebble or stone) on the wound and ask the casualty to grasp it firmly in his or her clenched fist. Tie the triangular bandage over the clenched fist as described above, then elevate and support the hand with an elevation sling (see page 88).

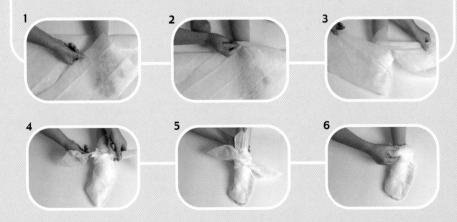

1 2 3 4 5 6

Applying a triangular bandage to a head

The scalp – the skin that covers the head – can bleed quite profusely if it is cut, often making an injury look more serious than it actually is. With all injuries to the head, a casualty must nevertheless receive medical attention to rule out the possibility of concussion or a skull fracture. Following a blow to the head, if the casualty becomes unconscious at any time, even for a short period, you must follow the ABC routine – check the airway, breathing and circulation – and should be prepared to resuscitate if necessary. Then continue to monitor the ABC and the casualty's responses until the emergency services arrive.

Triangular bandages are applied to the scalp to hold dressings in place. (Because they do not put pressure on a wound, they are not used for controlling bleeding.)

1 Fold a hem along the long base of a triangular bandage. Place the bandage so that the centre of the hem is above the space between the casualty's eyebrows and the point and ends are hanging down behind the head.
2 Cross the ends of the bandage at the back of the head, about level with the lowest point of the ears.
3 Take the ends round to the front of the head, leaving the pointed end hanging down, but trapped under the crossed ends. Tie the ends on the forehead using a reef knot (see page 73).
4 Steadying the casualty's head with one hand, very gently pull down the pointed end of the bandage at the back of the head with the other hand to tighten the bandage.
5 Bring up the pointed end and secure it to the bandage on the crown of the casualty's head with a safety pin.

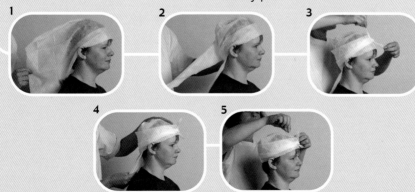

Slings

Two types of sling are made with triangular bandages: the arm sling and the elevation sling (also known as the St John sling).

A third sling, the collar-and-cuff sling, can be made either with a triangular bandage or with any suitable strip of clean fabric.

Applying an arm sling

The arm sling, which is used for injuries to the forearm and wrist, keeps the forearm in place across the casualty's chest. When correctly applied, the casualty's hand should be a little higher than the elbow, and the fingers – from the lower knuckles to the fingertips – should be clearly visible.

Before applying an arm sling, the casualty should be seated and, if possible, supporting the injured arm throughout the procedure, with his or her hand positioned a little higher than the elbow.

Place a triangular bandage over the casualty's chest. One point of the bandage should be pointing towards the elbow of the injured arm.

1 Gently slide the upper end of the bandage upwards, between the forearm and chest, making sure that the point at the elbow is level, but has some overlap.

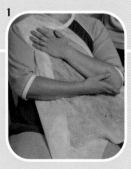
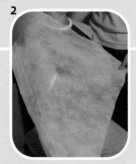

2 Bring the top point of the bandage over the shoulder on the uninjured side, round behind the neck and down over the shoulder on the injured side so that it lies in the hollow of the collarbone.

3 Bring the lower point of the bandage up, and over, the injured forearm.

4 Tie the two ends of the bandage together with a reef knot (see page 73) that lies in the hollow of the collarbone. Arrange the bandage so that the fingers are visible.

5 Bring the point of the bandage by the injured elbow across the forearm and secure it to the bandage with a safety pin. Check the casualty's circulation with a fingernail test (see page 73) and adjust the sling if necessary.

3
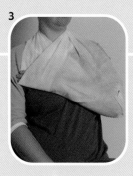

4
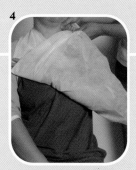

5
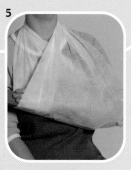

Dressings, bandages and slings

Applying an elevation (or a St John) sling

An elevation (or St John) sling is used to support the arm without putting pressure on an injured shoulder or collarbone. It is also used to support and raise a bleeding hand. When applied correctly, the hand should be in a raised position. The casualty should be seated and, if possible, supporting the injured arm throughout the procedure.

1 Arrange the casualty's injured arm naturally by his or her side, with the elbow bent and the forearm across the chest. The fingers on this hand should point to the opposite shoulder.

2 Place a triangular bandage over the forearm and hand, so that the one point of the bandage covers the elbow and there is plenty of overlap.

3 Gently pull the base point of the bandage under the forearm, elbow and hand.

4 Take the lower end of the bandage around the back and over the shoulder on the uninjured side and then adjust the height of the sling.

5 Tie the two pointed ends of the bandage together, as close to the fingers as possible, using a reef knot (see page 73).

6 Firmly tuck the loose point of the bandage near the elbow between the forearm and the front of the sling and then secure the fold to the sling with a safety pin.

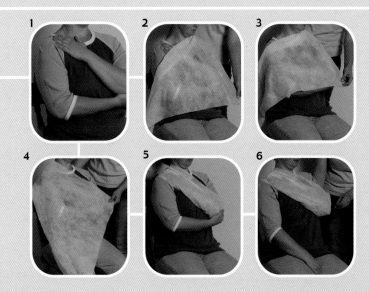

Applying a collar-and-cuff sling

The collar-and-cuff sling is useful when a casualty has either a fracture of the upper arm or an injured hand.
1 Using a bandage, or having folded a triangular bandage into a narrow one, form a clove hitch by making two loops, one towards you and the other away from you.
2 Fold over one loop so that it lies on top of the other.
3 Slide the loops over the wrist of the injured arm.
4 Gently elevate the arm against the casualty's chest and tie the bandage's two loose ends together at the side of the neck with a reef knot (see page 73).

1
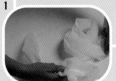

2
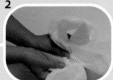

3
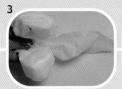

4
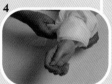

Improvised slings

If no bandages, triangular or otherwise, are available and the casualty's arm is not broken, you can fashion an improvised sling from the casualty's clothing.
a. If the casualty is wearing a pullover: with the casualty's hand held against his or her shoulder on the opposite side, support the arm by turning the hem of the pullover over it.
b. If the casualty is wearing a buttoned jacket or coat: place the casualty's hand inside his or her jacket or coat, fasten the lower buttons and then let the jacket bear the weight of the arm.
c. If the casualty is wearing a zip-up jacket: turn one side the front of the unzipped jacket over the injured arm and pin the hem to the front of the jacket with a safety pin. Alternatively, pin the sleeve's cuff to the lapel with a safety pin.

b
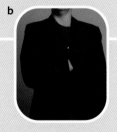

c
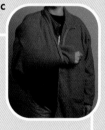

Dressings, bandages and slings

Chapter 4

Major injuries and serious conditions

In an emergency or at an accident site, after the first-aider has assessed the danger, checked the casualty's response, followed the ABC procedure – checking the airway, breathing and circulation (pulse) – managed life-threatening problems and called for medical assistance, an orderly assessment of the casualty can be undertaken.

The casualty should be examined for bleeding (internal and external bleeding, see pages 95 to 105), burns (see pages 108 to 116 and fractures (see pages 134 to 151), with any tenderness, swelling, wounds or deformities also noted. Check the casualty's body in the following order:

· the head and neck;
· the chest, including the shoulders;
· the abdomen, including the pelvis;
· the upper limbs;
· the lower limbs;
· the back.

Shock

Outside medical circles, the word 'shock' is often used to describe 'a fright'. Clinical or surgical shock has nothing to do with fright, however: it is a serious, life-threatening condition that can occur after a serious injury or sudden illness has befallen a casualty.

Shock is a condition in which either the amount of fluid in the blood vessels is insufficient to fill them or the heart's output is not sufficiently high to maintain blood circulation. In both cases, the casualty's blood pressure drops and the supply of oxygen to the vital organs of the body – in particular the brain, heart and kidneys – is not enough to keep them functioning properly. The body begins to compensate by shutting down the arteries to the less vital parts of the body, such as the skin and intestines, but this compensation is limited.

The causes of shock are as follows.

· Blood loss as a result of either external or internal bleeding (see pages 102 to 105), when the volume of blood in the blood vessels becomes insufficient.

· Severe blood infection (septicaemia), which can cause the blood vessels to widen, leading to fluid from the blood leaking into the body tissues.

· Fluid loss caused by prolonged vomiting or diarrhoea, which takes fluid from the blood, in turn reducing the volume of blood.

· Burns, which can cause large quantities of fluid to be lost from the body, either from the surface or through the formation of blisters.

· Heart attack or heart failure, when the weakened heart muscles may not be able to maintain blood circulation.

The symptoms and signs of shock

Because shock occurs progressively, there may be little evidence of it immediately after a casualty has been injured. The first-aider must therefore be vigilant in constantly checking for the symptoms and signs of shock, which depend on:
· the severity of the casualty's injury;
· the continuation of fluid loss;
· the effectiveness of shock management.

The initial symptoms and signs of shock include:
· a pale face, fingernails and lips and cold skin caused by the body shutting down the blood vessels that supply the skin;
· a rapid pulse caused by the heart attempting to maintain blood circulation;
· a weak pulse caused by the heart's inability to beat strongly enough;
· faintness, dizziness, drowsiness, confusion and nausea caused by a reduced blood supply to the brain and muscles.

Signs of worsening or severe shock include:
· the extremities – the fingers, nails, toes and lips – becoming blueish in colour;
· severe breathlessness due to the blood containing insufficient oxygen;
· severe thirst due to the blood's fluid content having been reduced;
· possible loss of consciousness due to the reduced blood supply to the brain; if treatment is unsuccessful, death may occur.

Major injuries and serious conditions

First-aid action and shock management

The aims of first aid are to prevent the worsening of the casualty's shock and to make the best use of his or her limited circulating blood, as follows.

· ABC: follow the airway, breathing and circulation (pulse) procedure (see pages 38 to 40).

· Control any severe bleeding (see page 99).

· Call for urgent medical assistance and reassure the casualty. Keep talking to the casualty and record his or her responses. Stay alert for any signs of confusion, drowsiness, faintness or nausea.

· Do not move the casualty unless it is absolutely essential because this could cause further bleeding and aggravate his or her shock.

· Do not give the casualty anything to eat or drink.

· Do not allow the casualty to smoke.

· Unless either of them are fractured, raise the casualty's legs above the level of the heart by laying the casualty down and elevating the legs with a folded coat or blanket. Keeping the head low enables gravity to assist the flow of blood to the brain, while keeping the legs high encourages the blood to remain in the central area of the body.

· Loosen any tight clothing.

· Dress any wounds or burns.

· Cover the casualty with a coat or blanket.

· Monitor the ABC (airway, breathing and circulation) regularly.

· If the casualty seems likely to vomit, if breathing becomes difficult or if the casualty loses consciousness, place him or her in the recovery position (see pages 42 to 43).

· If the casualty's breathing ceases, start artificial respiration (AR, see pages 44 to 46) or cardiopulmonary resuscitation (CPR, see pages 47 to 53) as appropriate.

Bleeding

The adult body contains about 5 litres (9 pints) of blood, although the quantity varies according to the person's size. An adult can safely lose – or donate – 500 millilitres (about 1 pint) of blood. A child weighing 30 kilograms (66 pounds) has only about 2.5 litres (5 pints) of blood, while a baby or infant weighing around 6 kilograms (about 13 pounds) has only around 750 millilitres (about 1 pint) of blood, and the loss of 300 millilitres (about ½ pint) may result in the baby or infant's death.

Bleeding occurs when the blood vessels are cut or torn. It may be external and visible, or internal and invisible, although internal bleeding may be indicated by a large amount of swelling around the site of the injury or a high degree of tenderness around the abdomen.

There are three types of bleeding: arterial bleeding, venous bleeding and capillary bleeding.

Arterial bleeding

The arteries carry oxygen-rich blood from the heart around the body. Arterial blood is bright red and spurts from wounds in time with the heartbeat. If left uncontrolled, it can quickly lead to dangerous blood loss to the extent that circulation cannot be maintained. The only thing that takes priority over treating arterial bleeding is ensuring that the casualty can breathe freely; thereafter you should apply direct pressure to the wound.

Venous bleeding

The veins carry deoxygenated blood around the body back to the heart. Venous blood is darker, more purple in colour, than arterial blood and pours, rather than spurts, from a wound.

Major injuries and serious conditions

Capillary bleeding

The capillaries are small blood vessels that link the arteries and veins. If a capillary is cut or damaged, blood will ooze from it. The most common types of everyday wound produce this type of bleeding.

Controlling external bleeding

Severe bleeding is always serious and can be fatal, so act quickly and remember that the true extent of the bleeding may be hidden. Having assessed the scene for danger, checked the casualty's responses and followed the ABC (airway, breathing and circulation) procedure if necessary, calm the casualty. Ask him or her to sit down or, if the bleeding is severe, to lie down. If the bleeding is from a limb, raise the limb above the level of the casualty's heart and then support it.

1 Check the wound for embedded objects (see page 80). If there are none, put on a pair of gloves (if they are available) and either apply direct pressure to the wound with your fingers or hand or, if possible, ask the casualty to do so. If an embedded object is present, apply pressure to either side of the wound.

2 As soon as possible, place a sterile dressing – or a clean piece of cloth, such as a folded handkerchief – over the wound and then bandage it (see pages 71 to 72).

3 Check the casualty's circulation by either locating a pulse (3a) or pressing a finger- or toenail (3b) (see page 73) of the injured limb. Look for signs of shock (see pages 92 to 94). **4** Do not interfere with any dressings or bandages because this may disturb any clot that is beginning to form and make the bleeding worse. If the bleeding continues, put another pad of absorbent material on top of the original dressing and bandage and then apply another bandage. Remember, too, to:

· continue to monitor the casualty for shock;

· to raise and support the injured limb;

· to loosen any tight clothing;

· not to give the casualty anything to eat or drink and not to allow him or her to smoke.

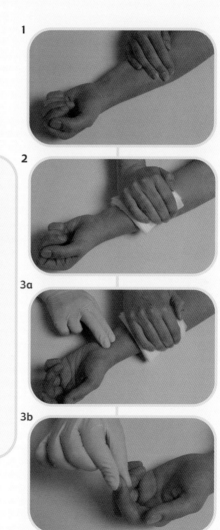

1

2

3a

3b

Major injuries and serious conditions

Uncontrolled bleeding

If, having applied direct pressure or a bandage, the bleeding will not stop and is severe, call for emergency medical assistance as a matter of urgency. You will then have to apply pressure to the artery leading to the wound to stop the flow of arterial blood. This is done by applying indirect pressure on the artery leading to the wound, at a point where the artery runs over a bone so that the artery is compressed between the fingers and the bone.

With the main artery to a leg or arm having been compressed in this way, the entire blood supply to the limb is cut off, and there is consequently a danger that the healthy tissue beyond the point of injury will be starved of circulating blood, causing the tissue to die and gangrene to set in. This is why stopping the flow of arterial blood should only be done when the situation is desperate.

The key points to remember are:

· that this procedure should only be used as a last resort;

· that the arterial blood supply must not be cut off for more than fifteen minutes at a time.

Arterial pressure points

The main artery in the arm runs down the inner side of the bone of the upper arm, and the location of the best compression point is about the middle of the bone of the upper arm.

The main artery of the leg enters the leg at about the middle of the fold of the groin. At this point, the artery runs over the bony ridge of the pelvis, and this is where the optimum pressure point is to be found.

Controlling severe bleeding: the arm

If a casualty's arm is bleeding severely, try to stem it in the following way.

1 Raise the casualty's injured arm above the head and locate the pressure point on the artery in the upper arm.

2 Compress the artery between your fingers and the arm bone, pressing firmly inwards and upwards between the arm muscles until you feel the bone and can see that the bleeding has been reduced.

3 Remember that you must not maintain pressure on the arterial pressure point for more than fifteen minutes. When the bleeding has been controlled, release the pressure from the pressure point and apply direct pressure to the wound.

4 Monitor the casualty's ABC (airway, breathing and circulation) and look for signs of shock.

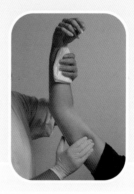

Controlling severe bleeding: the leg

If a casualty's leg is bleeding severely, try to control it as follows.

1 Lay the casualty on the ground, with his or her knees slightly bent, and locate the pressure point on the pelvic bone.

2 Using your thumbs or, if you are unsure of the exact location of the pressure point, the heel of your hand, apply pressure to the pressure point. (You will need to apply strong pressure in order to compress this major artery.)

3 Remember that you must not maintain pressure on the arterial pressure point for more than fifteen minutes. When the bleeding has been controlled, release the pressure from the pressure point and apply direct pressure to the wound.

4 Monitor the casualty's ABC (airway, breathing and circulation) and look for signs of shock.

Major injuries and serious conditions

Controlling severe bleeding: partial amputations

When a limb has suffered a major injury, as in the case of a partial amputation or shark attack, severe bleeding cannot always be controlled by applying direct pressure to the wound. Only in these circumstances may it be necessary to resort to applying a constrictive bandage above the casualty's elbow or knee until emergency medical assistance arrives.

1 Using a strip of firm cloth – either improvised from clothing or a narrow, folded triangular bandage – at least 7.5 cm (3 in) wide and 75 cm (30 in) long, bind the injured limb above the bleeding point until a pulse can no longer be felt beyond the constrictive bandage and the bleeding has been controlled. Firmly tie the bandage with a reef knot (see page 73).

2 Make a note of the time when you applied the constrictive bandage. After thirty minutes, untie the bandage and check for bleeding. If there is no bleeding, remove the bandage. If the bleeding recommences, apply direct pressure. If this is unsuccessful, reapply the constrictive bandage, make a note of the time and check for bleeding again after thirty minutes.

3 Monitor the casualty's ABC (airway, breathing and circulation) and look for signs of shock.

4 Make sure that the constrictive bandage is clearly visible and, when they arrive, inform the emergency services of its location and the time when it was applied.

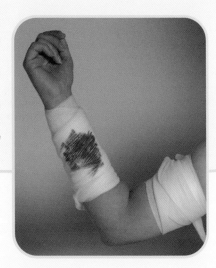

Controlling severe bleeding: severed body parts

If action is taken quickly enough, it may be possible to save a severed limb, finger or toe. The priority, however, is to save the casualty's life, so:

·call for emergency medical assistance as a matter of urgency;

· do not try to bandage a severed body part back in place because you will not only cause further distress, but will damage delicate tissues, which may hamper later microsurgery;

· be alert for signs of shock.

1 Lay the casualty on the ground and then support the injured limb in a raised position.

2 If they are available, put on a pair of gloves and then press a large piece of gauze or clean cloth firmly against the stump or raw area to control the bleeding before bandaging the dressing in place. Keep the casualty still and monitor him or her for signs of shock.

3 Find the severed body part and wrap it in a piece of sterile gauze or clean cloth; do not wash it. Place it in a watertight container, such as an inflated and sealed plastic bag, then place that into another container filled with water that is as cold as possible. (If ice has been added to the water, do not allow the body part to come into direct contact with it.) When the emergency services arrive, send the container to hospital with the casualty.

Major injuries and serious conditions

External bleeding and wounds

Minor wounds consist of abrasions and contusions.

· Abrasions are wounds to the surface of the skin caused by grazing or scraping. Subsequent bleeding is minimal.

· Contusions are wounds to, and below, the surface of the skin. Although bleeding is seldom severe, the skin may be split or bruised.

Minor bleeding does not often present any serious problems (unless the person affected is suffering from a disorder like haemophilia), but even small cuts and grazes may become contaminated with dirt or bacteria. (See page 125 for treating minor abrasions and contusions.)

By contrast, some types of wound can lead to severe and dangerous bleeding, particularly if an artery is cut. The open wounds listed below may also become infected and should always be examined by a doctor to avert serious or fatal infections.

· Incisions are cleanly cut wounds made by a sharp edge – a knife, for example. If the incision is in an artery, the bleeding may be severe and dangerous.

· Lacerations have 'torn', irregular edges and the bleeding can sometimes be severe.

· Penetrating wounds are serious and occur when an object penetrates the skin. Bleeding can be severe.

· Punctures have a small surface area, but may penetrate deep into the body. Bleeding may be a problem, particularly in the case of stab wounds, when serious or fatal internal bleeding may occur.

Puncture wounds may also lead to such dangerous infections as tetanus or gas gangrene.

. Perforating wounds pass right through the body, as with some stab or bullet wounds. Bleeding may be serious if an artery has been cut.

· Crater wounds occur when large amounts of tissue are suddenly torn from the body. Severe bleeding and shock may result.

In order to minimise the danger of infection when treating any such bleeding wounds, first-aiders should:

· wash their hands thoroughly both before and after administering first aid;
· handle a wound only when it is necessary to control severe bleeding;
· use sterile or clean dressings;
· avoid coughing, sneezing or talking when tending to a wound.

Clean the wound as thoroughly as possible.

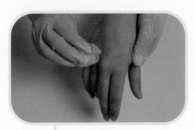

Managing incisions and lacerations

In the case of incisions and lacerations, after checking for danger, monitoring the casualty's response and following the ABC (airway, breathing and circulation) procedure, the first-aider should, if necessary:
· control the bleeding;
· clean the wound as thoroughly as possible;
· apply a sterile or clean dressing;
· seek medical assistance as a matter of urgency;
· reassure the casualty and make him or her as comfortable as possible.

Major injuries and serious conditions

Managing penetrating wounds

In the case of penetrating, puncture, perforating and crater wounds, after checking for danger, monitoring the casualty's response and following the ABC (airway, breathing and circulation) procedure, the first-aider should, if necessary:

· control the bleeding by applying direct pressure around the wound;

· cut, or otherwise remove, any clothing covering the wound;

· keep the wound as clean as possible; do not try to pick out any foreign material embedded in the wound;

· apply a sterile or clean dressing; in the case of a crater wound, it may be necessary to pack it with sterile or clean material and then apply direct pressure;

· seek medical assistance as a matter of urgency;

· reassure the casualty and make him or her as comfortable as possible.

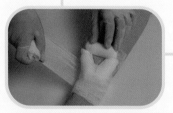

Where a foreign body is embedded, do not attempt to remove it, but bandage the wound using a ring padding.

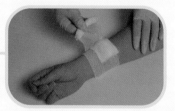

Control bleeding and apply a sterile or clean dressing.

Internal bleeding

The true extent of any severe bleeding may be hidden because it may be occurring internally. Internal bleeding may be difficult to detect, but should always be suspected if a casualty's injuries are severe, such as after a road traffic accident, or when a major bone, such as the femur (the thigh bone) or pelvis, has fractured, which may cause severe bleeding inside the body cavities. Severe bleeding is serious, and can be fatal, so act quickly.

The signs and symptoms of internal bleeding

The first symptom of internal bleeding is if the casualty is displaying signs of shock (see pages 92 to 94).

Suspect internal bleeding in the abdomen if:

· there is pain, tenderness and a large amount of swelling and extensive bruising around the site of the abdominal injury;

· the abdominal muscles are rigid.

Internal bleeding from some organs may be indicated if the casualty is:

· bleeding from an orifice, such as the mouth, nose or ears;

· vomiting either bright-red blood or blood the colour of coffee grounds (note that the blood may be mixed with food);

· coughing up red, frothy blood, in which case suspect an injury to the lungs;

· passing urine that has a red or smoky appearance, in which case suspect an injury to the bladder or kidneys;

· passing faeces that are red in colour, in which case suspect an injury to the small intestine;

· passing faeces that are black and tarry in appearance, in which case suspect an injury to the large intestine.

Managing internal bleeding

It is vital that you do the following when faced with a case of suspected internal bleeding:

· seek medical assistance as a matter of urgency;

· lay the casualty on the ground, unless he or she is coughing up red, frothy blood, in which case encourage the casualty to sit as comfortably as possible;

· raise the casualty's legs or bend the knees;

· check and record the casualty's circulation (pulse) every three to five minutes;

· reassure the casualty and monitor him or her for signs of shock;

· be prepared to administer AR or CPR if necessary (see pages 44 to 53);

· loosen any tight clothing;

· do not give the casualty anything to eat or drink, and don't allow him or her to smoke.

Major injuries and serious conditions

Crush injuries

Casualties sustain crush injuries when heavy weights fall on then, for example, when such major incidents as earthquakes occur, when buildings or other large structures collapse or when heavy objects, such as furniture, topple onto, and trap, a casualty.

Often characterised by fractures and open wounds caused by falling debris, further features of crush injuries affect the type of first-aid treatment that is administered: for example, crushed muscles release haemoglobin into the blood that can clog up the kidneys and prevent them from functioning, while bleeding into the muscles causes considerable blood loss.

In addition to an obvious heavy weight lying on, or across, a casualty, crush injuries are indicated by:
· severe swelling, bruising and blistering around the crushed area;
· the absence of a pulse (see pages 40 to 41) beyond the crushed area;
· cold and pale or discoloured limbs beyond the point of the crush injury;
· shock (see pages 92 to 94);
· fractures (see pages 134 to 151).

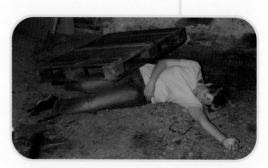

Before moving heavy objects off crush casualties first check that you will not cause further damage or injury by doing so.

The most practical and useful type of first-aid to administer depends on how long the casualty has endured the crushing force. If it is less than one hour, if possible, remove the crushing weight as fast as you can (but only if this will not further weaken an already damaged building or structure) and call for emergency medical assistance as a matter of urgency. Make a note of the length of time that the weight was crushing the casualty and when the casualty was released, and pass this information on to the emergency services when they arrive. The next steps are as follows.

1 Assess the casualty's injuries and ABC: airway, breathing and circulation (pulse). Do not allow the casualty to move. If the casualty is, or becomes, unconscious, place him or her in the recovery position (see pages 42 to 43).

2 Control any external bleeding (see pages 96 to 104).

3 Treat the casualty for shock (see pages 92 to 94).

If the casualty has been crushed under a heavy weight for more than one hour:

· call the emergency services as a matter of urgency and describe the incident clearly;

· do not remove the weight because this may cause even more serious injury;

· explain this to the casualty and reassure him or her;

· monitor the casualty's breathing and, if possible, ensure that the airway is kept open.

Major injuries and serious conditions

Burns

Burns can be caused by the dry heat of flames from a fire, but also by:
· hot objects, such as irons, saucepans, oven doors and car engines and exhausts;
· friction, such as that caused by a rope burn;
· chemicals, both acids and alkalis, which are present in paints, solvents and strippers and other substances, such as wet concrete and cleaning agents;
· electricity, from both domestic and high-voltage supplies;
· radiation, from the sun, sun lamps and microwaves;
· very low temperatures – liquid gases like nitrogen, as well as ice and ice-cold metal, can all cause 'cold burns'.

Scalds are caused by excessively hot steam or liquids. Both scalds and burns are serious injuries that may result in:
· the death of the superficial layers of skin or, in severe cases, the death of the entire skin structure and deeper tissues;
· damage to the superficial blood vessels, with outpourings of fluid causing blistering of the skin;
· a red-coloured, swollen, raw area that may become infected;
· severe pain;
· shock;
· in extreme circumstances, when the burns are deep or extensive, death.

Types of burn

The severity of a burn depends on the type and on the size of the area affected. There are three types of burn: superficial, intermediate (or partial thickness) and deep (or full thickness).

Superficial burns

Superficial burns affect only the epidermis (the top layer of the skin) and cause redness and swelling. Unless the affected area is extensive (see below), this type of burn is not serious, and if it receives immediate first aid, should heal within a few days without scarring.

Intermediate or partial-thickness burns

Intermediate, or partial-thickness, burns are deeper than superficial burns, affecting several layers of the epidermis and resulting in blisters. Although this type of burn usually heals, medical attention should be sought if the affected area is extensive (see below) or involves the face, hands or genitals.

Deep or full-thickness burns

Deep, or full-thickness, burns affect both the epidermis (the top layer of the skin) and the dermis (the underlying layer). They may also affect the nerves and tissues of a limb or adjacent organ. The burned area may look pale or charred, and the casualty may not feel any pain because the nerves have been damaged. Deep burns are often extensive and require medical treatment as a matter of urgency.

The burn area

The more extensive a burn – that is, the larger the area of the burn – the more serious it is likely to be. Shock (see pages 92 to 94) is the immediate threat to life caused by extensive burns; after forty-eight hours, the main danger is infection.

Even superficial burns can be dangerous if they are extensive, so ensure that any burn or scald that measures over 3 cm (1 in) is examined by a doctor.

An assessment of the seriousness of large burns is made using the 'rule of nines'. Each division of the human body as indicated on the diagram represents nine per cent of the body's total surface area. Any person with a burn – even a superficial burn – of more than nine per cent of the body area requires hospital treatment. The rule of nines is also used to assess the danger to the casualty's life and to determine the need for a blood transfusion or other type of transfusion.

Major injuries and serious conditions

Clothing on fire: stop, drop, wrap and roll

Many serious burns are caused by clothing catching fire, which often starts at the hem of a garment and may spread rapidly upwards if the casualty remains standing upright or, as is often the case, if his or her first reaction is to run around. If your clothes, or someone else's, are on fire, follow the stop, drop, wrap and roll procedure.

· **Stop:** because movement will fan the flames, keep the casualty still.

· **Drop:** tell the casualty to drop to the floor to prevent his or her face, neck and airway from being burned.

· **Wrap:** if there is no suitable dry-powder fire extinguisher to hand, smother the flames with a fire blanket or a piece of suitable heavy material (do not use nylon) to cut off the fire's oxygen supply.

· **Roll:** if no suitable smothering material is available, then, and only then, roll the casualty's burning side over the ground to extinguish the flames. (Rolling a casualty should only be a last resort because it may extend the burned area.)

Managing and treating high-temperature burns and scalds

If you are confronted by someone who has sustained high-temperature burns or scalds, immediately do the following.

· If the casualty has extensive burns, lay him or her down, but protect any burnt areas from direct contact with the ground.

· Be prepared to treat the casualty for shock (see pages 92 to 94).

· If the casualty has been in a fire – a house fire, for example – regularly check and monitor his or her breathing (see page 39) because the airway may have been damaged.

· As soon as possible, call for medical assistance as a matter of urgency.

Before administering first aid, assess the scene of the incident for danger.

· Remember that rescuing a casualty from a burning building can be dangerous and should be left to the experts whenever possible. Feel the temperature of the door, and if it is very hot, do not enter. If it is cold, or slightly warm, cover your mouth and nose with a damp cloth, crouch down low and open the door very slowly.

· If domestic-voltage electricity is involved, switch off the current or jerk the cable free (but do not cut it). If you cannot switch off the current and the casualty is still in contact with the electrical appliance and current, push clear any part of the casualty's body that is in contact with it, protecting yourself from the electrical current with the help of dry, non-conductive materials: a wooden broomstick while you stand on a dry rubber mat, a pile of newspapers or a telephone book, for instance.

· Note that if high-voltage electricity is involved – from overhead power cables, for example – it is normally fatal for the casualty. If they are within 18 metres (20 yards) of the electrical source, first-aiders may also be killed by 'arcing' or 'jumping' electricity. In such cases, call the emergency services immediately. You must keep clear of the area, and keep others away, until the current has been disconnected by the electricity-generating company. Do not touch the casualty, or any conducting material in contact with the current, until it has been disconnected.

Major injuries and serious conditions

3

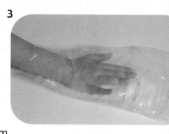

The aim in treating a burn or scald, be it minor or deep and extensive, is to reduce the effect of the heat on the skin, as well as to prevent infection from setting into the injured area.

1 Extinguish any burning clothes by smothering the flames with a blanket, jacket or dry-powder fire extinguisher.

2 Cooling the burns rapidly is now essential. Because hot clothing can itself cause serious burns, remove any such garments by cutting them off or dousing them with cold water. Keep cooling the casualty for the next ten minutes by pouring jugs or buckets of cold water gently over the burnt areas, but do not let this delay you from calling for emergency medical assistance to take the casualty to hospital. Do not overcool a serious burn either because this can cause hypothermia (see pages 202 to 203); shivering is a sign of overcooling.

3 While you are cooling the casualty, check his or her response (see page 37), constantly check the breathing (see page 39) and be prepared to resuscitate (see pages 44 to 53) him or her if necessary. If possible, remove any restrictive clothing or jewellery from the affected part of the body, but do not remove anything that is sticking to the skin.

4 Sit or lay the casualty down and constantly reassure him or her. Look for the signs of shock (see pages 92 to 94) and be prepared to treat it.

5 Cover the injury with a sterile dressing (see page 71). If no dressing is available, however, cover the burnt area with a clean polythene bag or clingfilm to reduce the risk of infection. Do not apply any lotions, ointments or any type of oily substance, including butter.

6 Keep checking the casualty's responses, breathing and circulation (pulse) until emergency medical assistance arrives. If the casualty is conscious and thirsty, frequently give him or her small sips of water.

Do not do any of the following:

· apply any type of lotion or ointment to a burn;

· prick or break any blisters (the outer layer of skin provides a perfect 'dressing' with which to protect the raw tissue below, which is prone to infection);

· give the casualty any alcohol to drink;

· overcool the casualty, especially if he or she is very young or the burnt area is extensive;

· directly apply towels, cotton wool, blankets or adhesive dressings to a burn.

Burns to the face and head

Burns to the face and head, as well as to the mouth and throat (which can be caused by overly hot objects, including food and drinks, or by inhaling hot gases or steam) can cause swelling that will rapidly block the airway. Immediate medical attention is therefore required.

Managing burns to the head

If the casualty has sustained burns to the head or face, take the following first-aid measures.

· Keep the burnt area cool by gently pouring cold water over it (use a jug or watering can).

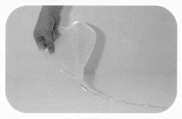

· Call for emergency medical assistance as a matter of urgency.
· Check the casualty's breathing and circulation (pulse) (see pages 38 to 41), look for signs of shock (see pages 92 to 94) and be ready to resuscitate if necessary (see pages 44 to 53).
· Do not apply a tight dressing to a head burn, but instead either use a triangular bandage (see page 85) or hold a dressing in place with your hands until emergency medical assistance arrives.

Major injuries and serious conditions

Managing burns in the mouth and throat

If he or she has been burned in the mouth or throat, a casualty will:

· be suffering great pain;

· be having difficulty breathing;

· often show visible signs of having been burnt, such as damaged skin, or even soot, around the mouth.

In such instances, the first-aider's priority should be to do the following.

· Obtain medical assistance as a matter of urgency; tell the emergency operator that you suspect burns to the airway so that the correct treatment can be prepared and be ready for use when the emergency services arrive.

· Keep the airway open (see page 38): if the casualty is unconscious, loosen any tight clothing around the neck, open the airway, check the breathing, place the casualty in the recovery position (see pages 42 to 43) and be prepared to resuscitate (see pages 44 to 53).

· Administer oxygen, but only if you are trained to do so.

Treating chemical burns

Chemical burns are often caused by strong acids, such as those found in car batteries, as well as by alkalis like powerful bleaches and caustic soda. Many domestic cleaning and DIY products are furthermore highly corrosive, and it's important always to read and observe the manufacturer's instructions regarding their storage, use and disposal. Because contact with corrosive chemicals can cause serious injuries to the skin and eyes, wear appropriate safety clothing (such as gloves, masks or eye-protectors) when indicated.

Treat a chemical burn as follows.

1 Flood the affected area with running water for at least twenty minutes to disperse the chemical and cool the affected site. Treat accidental splashes of corrosive chemicals to the eyes in the same way, but be careful not to let the water run down the casualty's face because this could spread the chemical over a wider area. If the chemical is a dry powder, brush it off with a soft brush before washing it away with running water.

2 Remove any contaminated clothing or footwear, taking care to avoid

contaminating yourself as you do so. Do not try to pick off any chemical contaminants that may be sticking to the casualty's skin.

3 Cover the burn with a sterile dressing (see page 71). Look for the signs of shock (see pages 92 to 94) and, if necessary, treat them. Then immediately seek medical attention.

Low-temperature burns

We usually associate burns with high temperatures, but it is possible to suffer a low-temperature burn when the skin adheres to extremely cold, smooth surfaces, such as a car's door handle in very cold weather conditions. Some gases, such as nitrogen, can be compressed and stored in liquid form at very low temperatures, and their leakage can also cause 'cold burns'.

Treating cold-burn injuries

Rather than cooling a cold burn, as you would for a high-temperature burn, it's important to raise the temperature of the skin to as near to normal body temperature as possible. The initial treatment should therefore be to wash the burn with lukewarm water, followed by treatment for frostbite (see pages 200 to 201). Medical attention should be sought for blistering.

Major injuries and serious conditions

Treating electrical burns

Electrical burns can occur when an electrical current passes through the body. A small burn may be evident at the point of contact, but electrical burns can also cause internal injury and lead to loss of consciousness. Seek medical attention for all such burns.

The first priority is safety: if the electrical current is domestic voltage, switch it off or break the casualty's contact with it (see page 111) before checking the casualty's response (see page 37). Do not approach a casualty who has sustained high-voltage electrical burns until the current has been switched off by the appropriate authority and keep at a distance of at least 18 metres (20 yards) to avoid being electrocuted by an 'arcing' current.

If the casualty is unconscious, open the airway, check the breathing and circulation (pulse) (see pages 38 to 41), move him or her into the recovery position (see pages 42 to 43) and be prepared to resuscitate (see pages 44 to 53) if necessary. Then do the following.

1 Having made sure that the casualty is no longer in contact with the electrical current, gently pour cold water over the burnt area. Then cut away any clothing around the burn.

2 Apply a sterile or clean, non-stick, non-fluffy dressing (see pages 68 to 72) to the burn; alternatively, use a clean plastic bag or a piece of clingfilm. If a hand or foot has been burnt, place it inside a clean plastic bag and secure it with some tape. Now call for emergency medical assistance.

3 Reassure the casualty and constantly check for signs of shock (see pages 92 to 94).

Angina, heart attack and cardiac arrest

Because the heart is responsible for keeping the blood circulating around the body, any problems experienced by this muscle can starve vital organs of essential oxygen.

Angina

Angina (*angina pectoris*) is not a disease in itself, but a symptom of heart disease. It is the pain that originates when the heart is trying to work without sufficient oxygen and is often due to the narrowing of the coronary arteries by the disease atherosclerosis. Angina attacks, and the onset of pain, often occur after a certain amount of physical exertion, or when strong emotional reactions are being experienced, and are usually relieved by rest and medication.

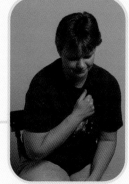

Those who have been diagnosed with angina, who are usually undergoing medical treatment, are likely to understand the nature of their condition and to carry medication for use during angina attacks.

Angina attacks often occur after physical exertion or when strong emotions are being experienced.

Major injuries and serious conditions

The signs and symptoms of angina

The symptoms of angina are pain and discomfort in the centre of the chest, which may radiate up the neck, into the jaw and down either arm, although it is commonly felt in the left arm. There may be breathlessness, a pallor of the skin and blueness of the lips.

The management of angina

When an angina attack strikes, the first-aider's aim should be to reduce the amount of work that the casualty's heart is being subjected to, as follows.

1 Do not let the casualty walk around. Help him or her to sit down and rest in the most comfortable position, using cushions, pillows or rolled-up clothes to support and bolster the casualty. Loosen any tight clothing and reassure the casualty.

2 Ask the casualty if he or she is carrying angina medication. If this is available, and in pill form, instruct the casualty to place the prescribed dose under his or her tongue or inside the cheek, depending on what the label indicates. If the medication is in spray form, administer it under the tongue.

3 Two or three minutes later, ask the casualty if the pain is passing. If it is persisting, the casualty may be suffering a heart attack (see below for treatment).

Heart attack

A heart attack is caused when a branch of a coronary artery becomes blocked and the part of the heart muscle that was previously supplied with blood by the blocked branch dies. The severity of a heart attack depends on the extent of the damage to the muscle: if a large area of heart muscle has died, a victim is unlikely to survive; if the area is small, recovery is possible, but the heart will be weakened by the dead area of muscle being replaced by scar tissue.

The signs and symptoms of a heart attack

The signs and symptoms of a heart attack are as follows:
· the sudden onset of a crushing pain in the centre of the chest, with the pain sometimes radiating outwards to the arms, back or throat;
· shortness of breath;
· faintness and sometimes loss of consciousness;
· nausea and sometimes vomiting;
· a pale, cold, clammy skin and profuse sweating;
· a weak, fast pulse that may also be irregular (an average healthy pulse is a steady 60 to 80 beats per minute);
· anxiety and distress – sometimes manifested by the casualty's conviction that he or she is dying – or confusion;
· sometimes an immediate collapse – cardiac arrest (see pages 120 to 121) – leading to the disappearance of the pulse.

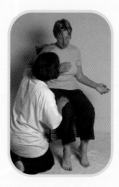

If you suspect a heart attack, help the casualty to sit down and keep him or her calm. Stay vigilant and follow ABC procedure.

Major injuries and serious conditions

Managing a heart attack

If you think that someone is having a heart attack, don't allow him or her to move around.

1 If the victim is conscious, help him or her to sit down, supporting the head, shoulders and bent knees with cushions, pillows or rolled-up blankets (this puts less strain on the heart than if the casualty were to lie down). Ask the casualty to relax. Now call for emergency medical assistance as a matter of urgency. Loosen any tight clothing at the neck, chest and waist.

2 Check the casualty's circulation (pulse) (see pages 40 to 41) and breathing (see page 39).

If the casualty loses consciousness, place him or her in the recovery position (see pages 42 to 43) and continue to monitor the breathing and circulation (pulse).

If the casualty's breathing stops, commence artificial respiration (AR, see pages 44 to 46).

If the casualty's heart stops (cardiac arrest, see below), commence cardiopulmonary resuscitation (CPR, see pages 47 to 53).

Cardiac arrest

Cardiac arrest is when the heart stops beating, either following a heart attack or as a result of other injuries or traumas.

The signs and symptoms of cardiac arrest

The signs and symptoms of cardiac arrest include when:
· the casualty collapses and becomes motionless and unconscious very quickly;
· there are no signs of breathing (see page 39);
· no pulse can be felt anywhere (see pages 40 to 41);
· the skin is grey in colour.

The management of cardiac arrest

If a casualty appears to have suffered cardiac arrest, do the following.
1 Call for medical assistance as a matter of urgency.
2 Begin artificial respiration (AR, see pages 44 to 46), giving two inflations of the casualty's chest by the 'mouth-to-mouth' method.
3 Begin cardiopulmonary resuscitation (CPR, see pages 47 to 53) and administer chest compressions.
4 Give two inflations after every fifteen compressions and continue doing so until help arrives.

Major injuries and serious conditions

Chapter 5

Bone, joint and muscle injuries

The bones of the skeleton are normally very strong, but can nevertheless break or fracture if struck, twisted or overstressed. Because the skeleton protects and surrounds important blood vessels, nerves and organs, skeletal injuries need to be handled very carefully in order to avoid causing further damage. The points at which the bones meet are the joints, which can be sprained or dislocated, while the muscles and tendons that move the bones can become strained.

Before treating any type of bone, joint or muscle injury, remember to:

· be aware of any danger, to check for hazards before doing anything else and not to approach a casualty if there is a danger to you;

· check the responses (see page 37) if the casualty is conscious;

· follow the first-aider's ABC – check the airway, breathing and circulation (pulse) (see pages 38–41) – and be prepared to resuscitate if necessary.

Injury management

If you think that someone has suffered a bone, joint or muscle injury, do the following.

1 Do not move the casualty unless he or she is in danger. If the casualty must be moved, however, support the injury throughout (see moving a casualty, pages 22 to 31, and step 3).

2 Call for emergency medical assistance.

3 Support and cushion the injured part, using both hands to support the injury above and below the joint and bolstering the injured area with pillows, if available, or rolled-up clothes.

4 Protect any open wounds from infection by covering them with sterile dressings or a piece of clean, non-fluffy material.

5 Look for, and be prepared to treat, shock (see pages 92 to 94).

Limb injuries

Injuries to the arms or legs can involve damage to the bones, joints, ligaments, muscles, major blood vessels and nerves. Depending on their severity, limb injuries can cause great pain and long-term disability and, in some instances, may even be potentially life-threatening: there may be blood loss from external wounds, as well as from internal injuries (especially in cases of multiple injury), for instance, while there is always a danger to the casualty's life due to shock (see pages 92 to 94).

Minor limb injuries

Minor limb injuries include cuts and grazes, friction burns, bruises and cramp.

Cuts and grazes and their treatment

This is the procedure for treating minor abrasions, such as small cuts and grazes.

1 Rinse the cut or graze under cold running water to remove any dirt.

2 Examine the wound for embedded objects (see page 80).

3 Wipe the area around the wound with sterile gauze swabs, cleaning from the wound outwards and using a fresh swab for each stroke.

4 Dry the wound with a sterile swab.

5 Apply an appropriate sterile dressing (see pages 71 to 72) to protect the wound from becoming infected.

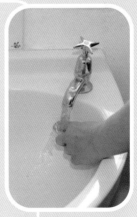

Whenever possible, wash your hands before treating any wounds.

Bone, joint and muscle injuries

Friction burns and their treatment

A friction burn occurs when the skin is rubbed against a surface. Such burns are most often experienced on the feet, particularly on the heel, after it has rubbed against a sock or shoe.

They can occur on other parts of the body, too: on the hands, after prolonged use of a hand tool, for instance; or on the inner thighs and underarms, often caused by clothes chafing while a person is jogging.

Treat a friction burn by cleaning the affected area and applying a sterile dressing (see pages 71 to 72). Do not prick or break any blister that forms because this protects the underlying raw skin from becoming infected. Procedure shown below.

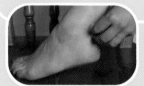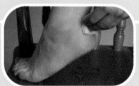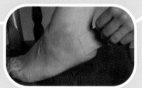

Applyling a sterile dressing to a friction burn.

Bruises and their treatment

Although a bruise may not appear for a day or so after the injury was incurred, the injury is often accompanied by immediate swelling. The aim of first aid is to minimise the swelling of the bruised area, and in the case of a bruised limb, the **RICE** procedure is the one to follow:

· **R:** rest the injured limb.

· **I:** apply an ice pack wrapped in a cloth to the injury. Place the ice pack on the affected part for twenty minutes, reapply it every two hours for the first twenty-four hours, then every four hours for the next twenty-four hours.

· **C:** apply either a compression bandage made of elasticated crêpe (see pages 74 to 77) or gentle pressure by compressing the injury with padding, such as cotton wool, and then securing the padding with a bandage (see page 72). The bandage should extend well beyond the injury.

· **E:** elevate the injured limb.

Ice packs and cold compresses

You can make an effective ice pack by filling a plastic bag two-thirds full with ice cubes and then squeezing out any remaining air and securing the top. Alternatively, simply use a bag of frozen peas. Such frozen compresses should be wrapped in a towel before being applied to an injury.

If an ice pack is not available, minimise the swelling of bruises or sprains, and thereby also the pain of the injury, by applying a cold compress and then supporting the injured part of the body in the position that the casualty finds the most comfortable. You can make a cold compress quickly and easily from a face flannel, a small towel or similar piece of material: soak it in cold water, wring it out, fold it to size and then place it over the injury. It can be resoaked every ten minutes or refreshed by gently dribbling cold water onto it. Compresses should be left on the injury for thirty minutes, either uncovered or secured in position with a bandage (but make sure that the bandage is not so tight that it restricts the circulation).

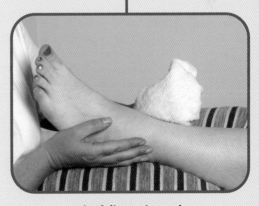

Applyling an ice pack.

Bone, joint and muscle injuries

Cramp and treatment

A common affliction of athletes and dancers, cramp is a sudden pain that is caused when a muscle, or group of muscles, contracts and tightens. Although initially painful, cramp can normally be relieved by stretching the affected muscles. If the sufferer has been sweating profusely from exertion or exercise, drinking a glass of water with a pinch of salt dissolved in it can also help (see also heat exhaustion, page 197).

a. Cramp in the hand is characterised by tight, bent fingers. Relieve the cramp by straightening the fingers and massaging the hand.

b. In the foot, straighten bent toes by gently pushing them upwards, towards the front of the leg, and then standing on the ball of the foot.

c. In the calf (lower-leg) muscle, straighten the knee and pull the foot up, towards the shin, as far as possible before massaging the calf muscle.

d. In the back of the thigh, support the leg and straighten the knee by pulling the leg gently up and forwards and then gently, but firmly, pressing the knee downwards.

The cramp that is commonly known as a 'stitch' in the side is often relieved simply by bending over at the waist and 'kissing' your knee. This is also a good method of relieving small children's abdominal cramp, especially if the pain has frightened them.

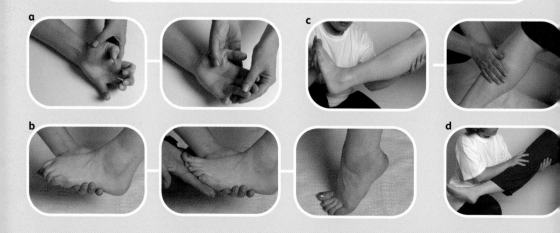

More serious limb injuries

More serious limb injuries include sprains, strains and dislocations.

Sprains
A sprain occurs when the ligaments that hold the bones together at the joints are stretched or torn. A sprain is a very painful injury, and is easily mistaken for a broken bone.

The signs and symptoms of a sprain

The signs and symptoms of a sprain are:
· intense pain;
· the injured part's restricted movement and loss of function;
· the inability of a sprained knee or ankle to bear the casualty's weight;
· swelling;
· bruising, which may develop quickly.

Treating a sprain

Because it may be difficult to tell the difference between a sprain and a fracture, the first-aider should approach, and manage, a sprain as if it were a more serious fracture. The first-aider should consequently:
· check for danger;
· check the casualty's response (see page 37);
· follow the ABC procedure – airway, breathing and circulation (pulse) (see pages 38 to 41) – and be prepared to resuscitate if necessary.

If the casualty is in great pain, or unable to move the affected limb, and you therefore suspect a serious injury, seek immediate medical attention because an X-ray diagnosis and specialist treatment may be required.

The aim of first aid is otherwise to reduce the swelling and pain by following the RICE procedure: rest, ice, compress and elevate (see also page 126).
1 Sit or lay the casualty down and rest the injured limb in a comfortable position.
2 Apply an ice pack or cold compress to the affected area to reduce the flow of blood and thereby minimise the subsequent swelling.
3 Compress the injury with some soft padding, such as cotton wool, secured with a bandage (see pages 68 to 72).
4 Elevate and support the injured limb to minimise bruising. If the wrist, arm or elbow is sprained, support the affected arm with an arm sling (see pages 86 to 87) and then seek medical attention.

1
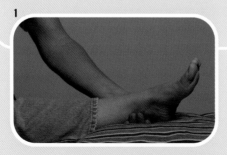

4
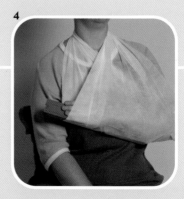

Strains

A strain occurs when a sudden movement or violent contraction tears a muscle or tendon.

The signs and symptoms of a strain

The signs and symptoms of a strain include:
· the sudden onset of pain – usually sharp pain – in the affected region;
· additional pain on moving or if the affected muscle is stretched;
· a loss of power in the affected region;
· the tenderness of the affected muscle;
· sometimes a gap in the muscle.

Treating a strain

Because it may be a more serious injury, before treating a strain, approach the casualty with care:
· check for danger;
· check the casualty's response (see page 37);
· follow the ABC procedure – airway, breathing and circulation (pulse) (see pages 38 to 41 – and be prepared to resuscitate if necessary;
· if necessary, get medical attention for the casualty.
  The aim of first aid is to reduce the swelling and pain, as follows.
1 Apply a cold compress to the injured area and advise the casualty not to stretch the muscle too much.
2 Support the injured muscle by applying a compression bandage (see pages 74 to 77).
3 Encourage the casualty to take very gentle exercise to reduce any painful spasms and shortening of the muscle. Do not rub or massage the injured area.

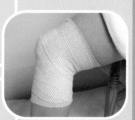

Treat a sprain with a cold compress and a compression bandage.

Bone, joint and muscle injuries

Dislocations

A dislocation of a joint occurs when an external force stretches the ligaments so far that the bones in the joint are pushed into an abnormal relationship, that is, out of their normal contact with each other. Some dislocations occur because the joint tissues are abnormally lax (loose), while others may involve either tearing of the soft tissues (ligaments and joint capsules) or a fracture of the bone (see pages 134 to 137). The most common dislocations are to the shoulder, jaw and thumb.

The signs and symptoms of a dislocation

The signs and symptoms of a dislocation include:

· severe pain, except when previous dislocations have previously occurred;
· deformity, that is, if the joint has an abnormal shape and appearance when compared to its 'twin' on the other side of the body;
· tenderness around the affected joint;
· the rapid development of swelling and bruising around the affected joint;
· an inability to move the affected joint.

Managing a dislocation

If the first-aider is in any doubt as to the nature of the injury, he or she should regard it as if it were a fracture (see pages 134 to 137), approach the casualty with care and:
· check for danger;
· check the casualty's response (see page 37);
· follow the ABC procedure – airway, breathing and circulation (pulse) (see pages 38 to 41) – and be prepared to resuscitate if necessary;
· if necessary, get medical attention for the casualty.

Do not attempt to treat the dislocation by moving or 'clicking' the bones back into position because doing this could damage the surrounding tissues and nerves and, in the case of a fracture, make it worse.

Do not give the casualty any food or drink because a dislocation may need to be treated in hospital under general anaesthetic.

1 Help the casualty into a position that he or she finds comfortable and offer reassurance. Check the circulation (pulse) in the affected limb (see pages 40 to 41). If it is undetectable, gently move the limb to restore the circulation and call for medical assistance.

2 Support the affected joint with pillows, rolled-up blankets or clothes in the position in which it was found and apply cold compresses or ice packs, and call for medical assistance.

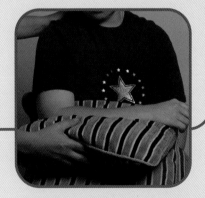

Support the affected joint in the position in which it was found.

Bone, joint and muscle injuries

Fractures

A fracture occurs when a forceful impact breaks or cracks a bone, or when a bone is bent or twisted. Fractures can also be caused when muscles exert excessive stress on bones (this commonly occurs when elderly people, for example, trip and try to prevent themselves from falling, the sudden contraction of a muscle thus causing a fracture) or when bones are weakened by disease. Not only do old bones break more easily than young ones, they also break more cleanly. Young bones can often bend without breaking completely: this is called a 'greenstick' fracture. Fractures of large bones can result in severe bleeding, both internal and external bleeding (see pages 95 to 105). A fractured thigh, for instance, may result in the loss of 1 to 2 litres (34 to 68 fluid ounces) of blood.

The three main types of break are closed fractures, open fractures and complicated fractures.

Closed fractures

A closed fracture is characterised by unbroken skin, that is, the broken part of the bone has not protruded through it. Although there is no external wound or bleeding, internal bleeding (see pages 104 to 105) does occur into the tissues.

Open fractures

When the bone protrudes through the skin, it is an open fracture. Blood loss may be severe and the open wound can become infected.

Complicated fractures

Complicated fractures may damage vital organs: a rib fracture (see chest injuries, pages 172 to 177), for example, may injure the lung.

The signs and symptoms of a fracture

The signs and symptoms of a fracture are as follows:
· the break may be felt or heard;
· intense pain is experienced around the site of the break;
· deformity of the affected limb, such as an abnormal twisted position or shortening;
· painful, difficult or impossible normal movement of the affected limb;
· a loss of power;
· tenderness when gentle pressure is applied to the affected area;
· swelling over, and possibly around, the fracture;
· bruising;
· in an open fracture, visible external bleeding;
· possible shock (see pages 92 to 94);
· crepitus: a grating sensation and sound as one end of the broken bone moves against the other.

Fractures: the rules

If you think that someone has suffered a fracture, it is vital that you observe the following rules.
· Do not test for crepitus because this may cause further injury.
· Do not move the casualty unless it is absolutely essential (see pages 22 to 31 on moving a casualty) because you will be putting him or her in further danger, particularly if you suspect neck or spinal injuries (see pages 152 to 154).
· Do not give the casualty any food or drink because a general anaesthetic may need to be given.
· Call for emergency medical assistance immediately.

Bone, joint and muscle injuries

Managing fractures: general principles

These are the general first-aid principles for managing a fracture.

· Assess the scene for danger and check the casualty's response (see page 37).
· If necessary, follow the ABC procedure – airway, breathing and circulation (pulse) (see pages 38 to 41) – and be prepared to resuscitate (see pages 44 to 53).
· Look for signs of shock (see pages 92 to 94) and be prepared to treat it.
· Control any bleeding (see pages 95 to 105) and dress all wounds (see pages 68 to 72).
· Check the circulation (pulse) beyond the fracture site; if there is no pulse, treat the situation as an urgent emergency and call an ambulance.

While you are waiting for medical assistance, follow the next steps.
1 Ask the casualty to sit or lie still and make him or her as comfortable as possible.
2 Steady and support the injured area by placing your hands above and below the point of injury. Reassure the casualty.
3 Continue to be alert for signs of shock, and if the casualty goes into shock, treat him or her accordingly (see pages 92 to 94), taking care not to move the injured joint.

Open fractures

With open fractures, there is always a wound near the fracture site. The protruding end of the broken bone may also be visible.

1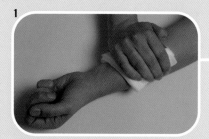

If the fractured bone is not protruding:
· assess the scene for danger and check the casualty's response (see page 37);
· if necessary, follow the ABC procedure – airway, breathing and circulation (pulse) (see pages 38 to 41);
· call for emergency medical assistance;
· be prepared to resuscitate (see pages 44 to 53 if necessary;
· look for signs of shock (see pages 92 to 94) and be prepared to treat it.

Then take the following steps.
1 If there is a lot of bleeding, try, if possible, to control the bleeding (see pages 95 to 105) by applying pressure and squeezing the edges of the wound together.
2 Cover the wound with a sterile dressing or pad of clean material, such as a folded handkerchief.
3 Secure the dressing with a pad of cotton wool or another type of soft, non-fluffy, non-adhesive material and then bandage the dressing in place (see page 72). Do not tie the bandage too tightly in case you impair the circulation.
4 Keep the injured limb still by supporting it fully and securely with your hand until the casualty can be transported to hospital.

If the fractured bone is protruding:
· assess the scene for danger and check the casualty's response (see page 37);
· if necessary, follow the ABC procedure – airway, breathing and circulation (pulse) (see pages 38 to 41);
· call for emergency medical assistance;
· be prepared to resuscitate (see pages 44 to 53) if necessary;
· look for signs of shock (see pages 92 to 94) and be prepared to treat it.

Then take the following steps.
1 Place a sterile gauze dressing or piece of clean, non-fluffy, non-adhesive cloth over the wound.
2 Place a ring bandage (see page 82) around the open wound or else pad it out with 'sausages' of cotton wool or rolls of bandage. The ring bandage or padding must be higher than the protruding bone.
3 Secure the ring bandage in place with diagonally placed bandages (see page 81).
4 Keep the injured limb immobile by supporting it fully and securely with your hand until the casualty can be transported to hospital.

4

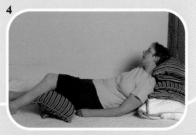

Bone, joint and muscle injuries

Immobilising a fracture

Paramedic ambulance crews will be equipped with splints with which to immobilise a fracture. If you must apply an emergency splint – perhaps because the casualty must be moved away from further danger – remember the following:

· splints must prevent any movement in both the joint above and the joint below the site of the fracture;

· the fracture site must be carefully padded to avoid any undue pressure being put on it, that is, unless it is necessary to control severe bleeding (see pages 99 to 101);

· fractures of the arm, hand or collarbone can be made more comfortable with padding and a sling (see pages 86 to 89);

· neck or spinal injuries are dangerous and must be handled with great care: do not move a casualty with suspected neck or spinal injuries unless it is absolutely necessary to remove him or her from danger.

Bandages and splints can both be used to immobilise a fracture.

Bandages

Observe the following rules when using bandages to immobilise a fracture:

· use broad bandages whenever possible;

· support the affected limb until the bandages are securely in place;

· gently pass the bandages under the natural hollows of the body, such as behind the ankles, knees or the hollow of the back;

· check the bandages to ensure that they are not so loose that they either slip or fail to support the fracture;

· check the bandages every fifteen minutes to ensure that they are not too tight.

Splints

Before applying a splint to a fracture, note the following advice:

· a splint must be both rigid and long enough to extend beyond the joints at either end of the fractured bone;

· padding should be placed between the splint and the natural curves of the body;

· place bandages at each end of the affected limb, just above and just below the fracture; secure the furthest bandage first, then the bandage at the other end of the limb, followed by bandages above and below the fracture site, thereby securing the splint against the padding applied to the injured limb.

· secure bandages on the casualty's uninjured side with a reef knot (see page 73).

The signs and symptoms of a fractured collarbone

If any of the following apply, the casualty may have a fractured collarbone:

· if he or she has a history of a previous fall onto the outstretched arm or elbow;

· if he or she heard or felt the break occurring;

· if movement of the affected shoulder aggravates the pain;

· if the casualty is supporting the affected arm at the elbow and is inclining his or her head towards the injured side;

· if the shoulder appears lower on the uninjured side;

· if there is tenderness and swelling around the collarbone;

· if the casualty is showing signs of shock (see pages 92 to 94).

Bone, joint and muscle injuries

Managing a fractured collarbone

Before managing a fractured collarbone, do the following:

· assess the scene for danger and check the casualty's response (see page 37);

· if necessary, follow the ABC procedure – airway, breathing and circulation (pulse) (see pages 38 to 41);

· call for emergency medical assistance;

· be prepared to resuscitate (see pages 44 to 53) if necessary;

· look for signs of shock (see pages 92 to 94) and be prepared to treat it;

· control any bleeding (see pages 95 to 105) and dress any wounds (see pages 68 to 72).

Then take the following steps.

1 Help the casualty to position the arm on the injured side so that the fingertips rest on the opposite shoulder and the arm is supported at the elbow.

2 Support the casualty's arm in an elevation (or St John) sling (see page 88). Try not to move the arm excessively.

3 To make the casualty more comfortable, place some soft padding – a folded towel, for example – between his or her upper arm and chest.

4 Secure the elevation sling to the casualty's chest by arranging a broad bandage (see page 83) over the sling and around the body. Check the circulation (pulse) in the thumb (see page 73).

3
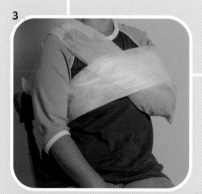

4
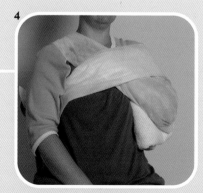

The signs and symptoms of a fractured upper arm

A fractured upper arm may be indicated by:

· a history of a fall onto, or pressure applied to, the affected arm;
· the break having been heard or felt;
· deformity, that is, an abnormal twisting or shortening, of the affected arm;

· painful, difficult or impossible normal movement of the affected arm;
· a loss of power and function in the affected arm;
· swelling of the affected arm;
· the casualty supporting the injured arm below the fracture site;
· possible signs of shock (see page xx).

Managing a fracture of the upper arm

Before treating a fracture of the upper arm:
· assess the scene for danger and check the casualty's response (see page 37);
· if necessary, follow the ABC procedure – airway, breathing and circulation (pulse) (see pages 38 to 41);
· call for emergency medical assistance;
· be prepared to resuscitate (see pages 44 to 53 if necessary;
· look for signs of shock (see pages 92 to 94) and be prepared to treat it;
· control any bleeding (see pages 95 to 105) and dress any wounds (see pages 68 to 78).
If the injury is not close to the elbow, do the following.

1 Sit the casualty down. Then bend, but do not force, the affected arm so that it lies across the torso. Pad the area between the fracture site and the casualty's chest with a folded towel or jumper.
2 Support the casualty's arm in a collar-and-cuff sling (see page 89).
3 Immobilise the arm with two broad bandages, one above the fracture around the arm and chest, the second below the fracture. Tie off the bandages with a reef knot (see page 73) at the front, on the casualty's uninjured side. Now check the circulation (pulse) (see page 40).

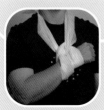 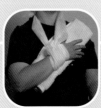 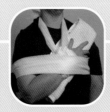 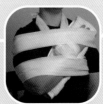

Immobilising the fractured arm

Bone, joint and muscle injuries

The signs and symptoms of a fractured forearm

A fractured forearm may be indicated by:
· a history of a fall onto, or pressure applied to, the affected arm;
· the break having been heard or felt;
· deformity, that is, an abnormal twisting or shortening, of the affected arm;
· painful, difficult or impossible normal movement of the affected arm;
· a loss of power and function in the affected arm;
· swelling of the affected arm;
· the casualty supporting the injured arm below the fracture site;
· possible signs of shock (see pages 92 to 94).

Managing a fracture of the forearm

Regardless of where the fracture has occurred, never forcibly bend a fractured forearm.

If the fracture is not near the elbow, first do the following:
· assess the scene for danger and check the casualty's response (see page xx);
· if necessary, follow the ABC procedure – airway, breathing and circulation (pulse) (see pages 38 to 41);
· call for emergency medical assistance;
· be prepared to resuscitate (see pages 44 to 53) if necessary;
· look for signs of shock (see pages 92 to 94) and be prepared to treat it.
The next steps are as follows.

1 Sit the casualty down and then immobilise the forearm firmly with a splint extending from the elbow to the fingers. Now bandage the splint in place as follows:
· above the fracture, below the elbow;
· below the fracture;
· at the wrist or hand.
2 Place the splint-encased arm in an arm sling (see pages 86 to 87) and then check the circulation and note the colour of the fingers by doing the fingernail test (see page 73).

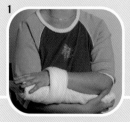
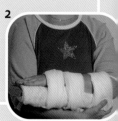

If the fracture is near the elbow, do the following.

· assess the scene for danger and check the casualty's response (see page 37);
· if necessary, follow the ABC procedure – airway, breathing and circulation (pulse) see pages 38 to 41;
· call for emergency medical assistance;
· be prepared to resuscitate (see pages 44 to 53) if necessary;
· look for signs of shock (see pages 92 to 94) and be prepared to treat it.

The next steps are as follows.

1 Lay the casualty down on their uninjured side, supporting the injured arm. Pad out the natural hollows of the casualty's body – for example at the waist. Do not bend the elbow, but gently place or slide a splint between the padding and the injured arm.

2 Immobilize the injured arm against the splint and body with broad bandages tied in front of the uninjured side.

1
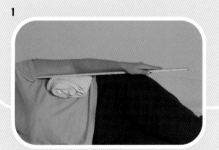

2
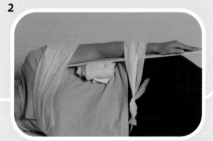

Fractures of the hands and fingers

Fractures of the bones of the hands and fingers are often the result of crushing. You may have to administer first aid for an open fracture (see page 137) and bleeding (see pages 95 to 105).

Bone, joint and muscle injuries

The signs and symptoms of a fracture of the hand or finger

The signs and symptoms of a fracture of the hand or finger include:
· a history of a fall onto, or pressure applied to, the affected hand or finger;
· the break having been heard or felt;
· deformity, that is, an abnormal twisting or shortening, of the affected hand or finger;
· painful, difficult or impossible normal movement of the affected hand or finger;
· a loss of power and function in the affected hand or finger;
· swelling of the affected hand or finger;
· possible bleeding (see pages 95 to 105);
· possible shock (see pages 92 to 94).

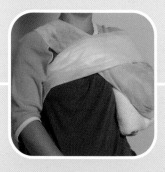

Managing a fracture of the hand or finger

Before managing a fracture of the hand or finger:

· assess the scene for danger and check the casualty's response (see page 37);
· if necessary, follow the ABC procedure – airway, breathing and circulation (pulse) (see pages 38 to 41);
· call for emergency medical assistance;
· be prepared to resuscitate (see pages 44 to 53) if necessary;
· look for signs of shock (see pages 92 to 94) and be prepared to treat it.
    After that, do the following (demonstrated above).
1 Sit the casualty down, remove any jewellery if possible, and then raise the affected hand to minimise any bleeding and swelling. Control any bleeding (see pages 95 to 105) and apply a pad and dressing (see pages 68 to 71) to the injured hand.
2 Place the injured arm in an elevation (St John) sling (see page 88) secured with a broad bandage (see page 83) applied over the forearm and around the casualty's chest and tied with a reef knot (see page 73) on the uninjured side.

The signs and symptoms of a fractured wrist

The signs and symptoms of a fractured wrist include:
· a history of a fall onto an outstretched hand;
· the break having been heard or felt;
· deformity, that is, an abnormal twisting or shortening, of the affected wrist;
· painful, difficult or impossible normal movement of the affected wrist;
· a loss of power and function in the affected wrist;
· swelling of the affected wrist;
· the casualty supporting the injured wrist;
· possible signs of shock (see pages 92 to 95).

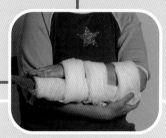

Managing a fracture of the wrist

Before managing a fractured wrist:
· assess the scene for danger and check the casualty's response (see page 37);
· if necessary, follow the ABC procedure – airway, breathing and circulation (pulse) (see pages 38 to 41);
· call for emergency medical assistance;
· be prepared to resuscitate (see pages 44 to 53) if necessary;
· look for signs of shock (see pages 92 to 94) and be prepared to treat it.

If the casualty is a child, he or she may prefer to support the fractured wrist him- or herself, which is fine. Otherwise follow these steps.

1 Sit the casualty down and rest the affected forearm and hand on a well-padded splint. Position additional padding under the hand and wrist if necessary.
2 Secure the arm to the splint with bandages (see page 139):
· below the elbow;
· across the back of the hand;
· around the middle of forearm.
3 If needed, elevate the affected arm and apply an arm sling (see pages 86 to 87). Now check the circulation (pulse) in the thumb (see page 73).

Bone, joint and muscle injuries

Fractured thighs

Fractures to leg bones are serious injuries and require urgent medical treatment, not least because fractures of large bones can cause severe bleeding, both internal and external (see pages 95 to 105), and in the case of a fractured thigh, 1 to 2 litres (34 to 68 fluid ounces) of blood may be lost.

The signs and symptoms of a fractured thigh

The signs and symptoms of a fractured thigh include:
· severe pain at the site of the injury;
· tenderness and swelling at the site of the injury;
· a loss of power and function in the affected leg;
· deformity, and possible rotation, of the foot of the injured leg;
· possible shortening of the injured leg;
· shock (see pages 92 to 94).

Managing a fractures of the thigh

Before managing a fractured thigh:
· assess the scene for danger and check the casualty's response (see page 37);
· if necessary, follow the ABC procedure – airway, breathing and circulation (pulse) (see pages 38 to 41);
· call for emergency medical assistance;
· be prepared to resuscitate (see pages 44 to 53) if necessary;
· look for signs of shock (see pages 92 to 94) and be prepared to treat it.

Then control any bleeding (see pages 95 to 105 and apply a dressing (see page 71) to any open wound. If a casualty has been lying unattended on the ground for a long period, also manage any scalds to the skin from urine or faeces, clean and dry the skin if possible, and reassure the casualty.

The next steps are as follows.
1 Place some padding between the casualty's legs and then gently move the uninjured leg adjacent to the injured leg.
2 Wind a figure-of-eight bandage (see page 83) around the casualty's ankles and feet.
3 Apply broad bandages (see page 83) around the knees and tie them with a reef knot (see page 73) on the uninjured side. Finally, check the circulation (pulse, see page 40 to 41).

1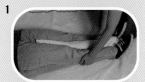

2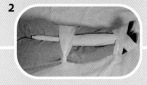

Fractured kneecaps

A kneecap can be broken by a direct blow or be split if the upper-leg muscles attached to it are violently pulled. Because it is difficult to distinguish between a broken kneecap and injury or damage to the cartilage or ligaments, all knee injuries should be approached as though they were fractures.

Bone, joint and muscle injuries

The signs and symptoms of a fractured kneecap

The signs and symptoms of a fractured kneecap are as follows:
· a history of a fall onto, or pressure applied to, the knee; pain over the kneecap that is aggravated by movement;
· deformity of the kneecap: sometimes a gap can be detected at the front of the knee or a displacement can be felt;
· an inability to straighten the affected leg;
· swelling and tenderness over the affected kneecap;
· possible shock (see pages 92 to 94).

Managing a fractured kneecap

Before treating a fractured kneecap:
· assess the scene for danger and check the casualty's response (see page 37);
· if necessary, follow the ABC procedure – airway, breathing and circulation (pulse) (see pages 38 to 41);
· call for emergency medical assistance;
· be prepared to resuscitate (see pages 44 to 53) if necessary;
· look for signs of shock (see pages 92 to 94) and be prepared to treat it;
· do not attempt to straighten the affected knee.

1 Lay the casualty on his or her back with the head and shoulders raised. Support and steady the injured leg in the position that the casualty finds the most comfortable by propping pillows, rolled-up blankets or clothes under, and around, the knee.
2 Although bandaging the injured kneecap is not essential, the casualty may find it more comfortable, in which case wind a figure-of-eight pressure bandage (see page 83) around the knee using a crêpe or conforming bandage (see pages 74 to 79), making allowances for any swelling.

1
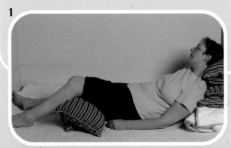

A fractured lower leg

When broken, the shinbone, which lies just below the skin at the front of the leg, can puncture the skin as described for an open fracture (see page 137).

The signs and symptoms of a fractured lower leg

The signs and symptoms of a fractured lower leg are as follows:
· a history of a fall onto, or pressure applied to, the affected leg;
· the break having been heard or felt;
· deformity, that is, an abnormal twisting, rotation or shortening, of the affected leg;
· a loss of power and function in the affected leg, including an inability to walk, or bear weight, on it;
· swelling of the affected leg;
· a bone protruding through the skin of the affected leg;
· bleeding;
· possible shock (see pages 92 to 94).

Managing a fracture of the lower leg

Before treating a fracture of the lower leg:
· assess the scene for danger and check the casualty's response (see page 37);
· if necessary, follow the ABC procedure – airway, breathing and circulation (pulse) (see pages 38 to 41);
· call for emergency medical assistance;
· be prepared to resuscitate (see pages 44 to 46) if necessary;
· look for signs of shock (see pages 92 to 94) and be prepared to treat it.
   Control any bleeding (see pages 95 to 105), apply a dressing to any open wound (see pages 68 to 72) and then do the following.

1 Place some padding between the casualty's legs and then move the uninjured leg adjacent to the injured leg, all the while supporting and steadying the injured limb.
2 Wind a figure-of-eight bandage (see page 83) around the ankles and feet and a broad bandage (see page 83) around the knees. Tie the bandages with reef knots (see page 73) on the casualty's uninjured side.

Bone, joint and muscle injuries

A fracture of the ankle

Note that it is often difficult to distinguish between an ankle fracture and a sprain (see page 129), especially if no deformity is visible.

The signs and symptoms of a fractured ankle

The signs and symptoms of a fractured ankle are as follows:
· a history of a twisting injury to the affected ankle;
· pain and swelling on either, or both, sides of the affected ankle;
· an inability to bear weight on the affected ankle;
· tenderness, especially on the bony 'peaks' on either side of the affected ankle;
· possible deformity, which may be severe;
· possible shock (see pages 92 to 94).

Managing a fracture of the ankle

Before managing a fracture of the ankle:
· assess the scene for danger and check the casualty's response (see page 37);
· if necessary, follow the ABC procedure – airway, breathing and circulation (pulse) (see pages 38 to 41);
· call for emergency medical assistance;
· be prepared to resuscitate (see pages 44 to 53 if necessary;
· look for signs of shock (see pages 92 to 94) and be prepared to treat it.

If there is no deformity, follow the RICE procedure (see page xx) and avoid placing any weight on the affected ankle until medical assistance arrives.
If there is deformity of the ankle, sit or lie the casualty on the ground, with the back and shoulders raised and supported. Support and steady the injured limb by resting it on a pillow or rolled-up blanket while you wait for the emergency services to arrive. Do not wind any compression bandages around the ankle.

The signs and symptoms of fractures of the feet or toes

The signs and symptoms of a fracture of the foot or toe include:
· pain;
· an inability to walk;
· tenderness and swelling;
· possible shock (see pages 92 to 94).

Managing a fracture of the foot or toe

Before managing a fracture of a foot or toe:
· assess the scene for danger and check the casualty's response (see page 37);
· if necessary, follow the ABC procedure – airway, breathing and circulation (pulse) (see pages 38 to 41);
· call for emergency medical assistance;
· be prepared to resuscitate (see pages 44 to 53) if necessary;
· look for signs of shock (see pages 92 to 94) and be prepared to treat it.

Do not remove the casualty's shoes and socks unless there is an open wound (see removing clothing, page 34).

If the casualty is not wearing shoes, do the following.

1 Apply a compression bandage (see pages 74 to 79) to the injured foot.

2 Raise the injured foot and rest it on a pillow or rolled-up blanket until medical assistance arrives.

Bone, joint and muscle injuries

Spinal injuries

Like head injuries, spinal injuries should always be regarded as serious, and if the casualty is unconscious as a result of a head injury, suspect a spinal injury. Spinal injuries require very careful management because if the casualty is moved unnecessarily, or handled incorrectly, the injuries may be aggravated and paralysis, or even death, may result, so do not move a casualty unless it is absolutely essential.

If you are the first person to arrive at the scene of an accident, your careful assessment of the scene for danger (see pages 10 to 14) and management of the casualty will be vital.

The causes of spinal injuries

If any of the following have occurred, suspect that the casualty has incurred a spinal injury.

· If the casualty has been involved in a car, motorcycle or bicycle accident.

· If the casualty has sustained a heavy blow to the head or back, for example, while engaged in a sporting activity like diving, a water sport, a contact or a 'dangerous' or 'extreme' sport, such as bungee-jumping, white-water rafting, parachuting or paragliding, on- and off-piste skiing or snowboarding.

· If the casualty has landed heavily on his or her feet (perhaps after jumping, or falling from, a raised structure), back or buttocks (such as after falling or slipping).

The signs and symptoms of spinal injuries

The signs and symptoms of spinal injuries include:
· pain at, or below, the site of the injury;
· undetectable or altered sensations, such as tingling in the hands or feet;
· loss of movement, or impaired movement, below the site of the injury;
· swelling and tenderness over the site of the injury;
· unconsciousness following a head injury.

Managing spinal injuries

If the casualty is unconscious and you suspect that he or she has sustained a spinal injury:
· assess the scene for danger and check the casualty's response (see page 37);
· if necessary, follow the ABC procedure – airway, breathing and circulation (pulse) (see pages 38 to 41);
· call for emergency medical assistance;
· be prepared to resuscitate (see pages 44 to 53) if necessary;
· look for signs of shock (see pages 92 to 94) and be prepared to treat it;
· before turning or moving the casualty onto his or her side, but only if you have to, apply a cervical collar (or an improvised version made from a folded towel or newspaper secured with a bandage) to minimise any movement of the neck.

Bone, joint and muscle injuries

If the casualty is conscious and you suspect that he or she has sustained a spinal injury:

· reassure the casualty;

· call for medical assistance as a matter of urgency;

· loosen any tight clothing;

· do not move the casualty unless absolutely essential;

· support the casualty's head and neck by placing your hands on either side of the head until another type of support can be arranged (this is important if a casualty has been found in a sitting position, perhaps if they have been trapped in a motor vehicle following a crash);

· apply a cervical collar (or an improvised version made from a folded towel or newspaper secured with a bandage) to minimise any movement of the neck;

· if the casualty has sustained a spinal injury in a diving or water-sport accident, support him or her with a floatation device or surfboard until medical assistance arrives.

Head injuries

A blow to the head that is forceful enough to cause a contusion or open wound (see page 102 can cause a fracture (see page 134). It may also result in unconsciousness, followed by concussion, a short period of impaired consciousness.

Because damage to the skull or brain may have occurred, no head injury should be regarded as minor or dismissed lightly.

The signs and symptoms of concussion

The signs and symptoms of concussion are as follows:
· loss of consciousness, perhaps only momentarily;
· pale, clammy skin;
· shallow breathing;
· nausea or vomiting;
· dizziness;
· the casualty's inability to remember the incident or the events preceding it;
· double vision;
· headache;
· shock (see pages 92 to 94).

Managing concussion

If the casualty is conscious, do the following.

1 Make the casualty comfortable (even if he or she does not appear to have been injured, there may be a delayed reaction to the incident). Do not give the casualty anything to eat or drink.

2 Apply a cold compress (see page 127) to the affected area of the head and watch for signs of the casualty's condition worsening, such as loss of consciousness or complications (see page 156).

If the casualty is, or becomes, unconscious, suspect a spinal injury (see pages 152 to 154) and support the head and neck if he or she moves, or is moved.

1 Place the casualty in the recovery position (see pages 42 to 43). Then follow the ABC procedure: open the airway, check the breathing and then the circulation (pulse) (see pages 38 to 41.)

If the casualty remains unconscious for three minutes or more, call for emergency medical assistance and continue to monitor the airway, breathing and circulation.

If recovery is rapid, check the casualty's response and watch for signs of deterioration or complications (see page 156).

Bone, joint and muscle injuries

The signs and symptoms of complications

Immediate medical attention is required if the casualty shows any of the following signs:
· abnormal- or different-sized pupils;
· discolouration or bruising around the eyelids or in the white part of the eye;
·unusually slow circulation (pulse);
· blood or blood-stained fluid flowing from an ear or the nose;
· bleeding from the scalp (which indicates a possible open fracture, see page 137).

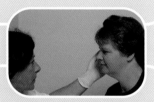

Managing complications

Manage a casualty who is displaying complications as if he or she were unconscious. Remember that because there is the possibility of a spinal injury (see pages 152 to 154), the head and neck must be supported if the casualty moves, or is moved. In addition, do the following.
· Place the casualty in the recovery position (see pages 42 to 43), check, clear and open the airway, monitor the breathing and then the circulation (pulse). If it is open, do not close the casualty's mouth and do not force open a clenched jaw.
· Control any bleeding (see pages 95 to 105), but do not apply direct pressure to the skull if you suspect that it has been fractured.
· If blood or fluid is flowing from an ear, lightly apply a sterile dressing (see page 71).
·Seek medical assistance as a matter of urgency.

Facial injuries

Because the eyes, nose and ears are located on the head, facial injuries can potentially result in such disabilities as the loss of sight, smell and hearing. These organs must therefore be protected following an accident, especially when a casualty is unconscious.

Eye injuries

The eyes are extremely delicate, sensitive and very susceptible to infection, which makes all eye injuries potentially serious, and medical treatment should therefore be sought as soon as possible to prevent permanent damage. Remember, too, to wash your hands if possible before administering first aid.

In the case eye injuries, both eyes need to be covered, which can be disorienting for a casualty, who will need your support and reassurance. If a casualty is wearing contact lenses and they can easily be removed from one or both eyes, ask him or her to remove them; do not attempt to remove a casualty's contact lenses yourself.

Bone, joint and muscle injuries

Black eyes and their treatment

A black eye is a bruise caused by a blow to the face that has injured the eyelid's thin, delicate skin, which covers many large veins. In most cases, little can be done apart from wait for the released blood to be reabsorbed, which can take between two and three weeks, and in the meantime watch the skin around the eye pass through a range of colours. Blows to the eye, or the area around the eye, can be more serious, however, because they could damage the eye or skull.

Treat a black eye as follows.

1 The sooner the eye area is cooled, the less swelling and pain the casualty will experience, so sit him or her down and place an ice pack (see page 127) on the eye area as soon after the injury has occurred as you can.

2 Remove the ice pack. Check the casualty's vision by gently pulling the affected eyelid slightly open with the forefinger and thumb of one hand and asking him or her to compare the vision in this eye with that of the unaffected eye. Ask the casualty to move the eye up and down and from side to side to check mobility, function and focus. If the casualty is experiencing any visual problems, he or she should be examined by a doctor.

Removing foreign objects from the surface of the eye

Tiny specks of dust, an eyelash or insect, cosmetics, grit, glass or metal particles can all cause considerable discomfort on the surface of the eye, including:

· pain in the eye, particularly when looking at the light;

· a watery, red eye;

· a partially, or completely, closed eye;

· spasms or twitching of the eyelid.

Before trying to remove a foreign object from the eye, note the following:

· do not attempt to remove a foreign object from the iris (the coloured part of the eye);

· do not let the casualty rub the affected eye;

· do not attempt to remove a foreign object that is embedded in any part of the eye;

· do not persist in examining an eye if the injury is severe.

A small foreign object may sometimes be washed out of the eye by the tears' natural action. If not, do the following.

1 Ask the casualty to look upwards. Gently draw the lower lid down and out. If the foreign object is visible, use the corner of a clean cloth moistened in water to remove it.

2 If the foreign object is not visible, ask the casualty to look downwards. Gently grasp the lashes of the upper lid and then pull the eyelid down and over the lower lid. This may dislodge the object.

3 If the foreign object still hasn't been dislodged, hold the eyelids apart and gently flush the eye with a weak stream of clean water.

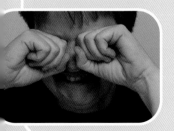

1

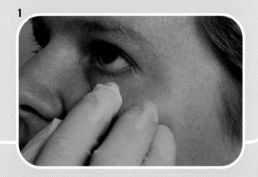

Bone, joint and muscle injuries

Managing wounds to the eye and embedded foreign objects

If the casualty has sustained a wound to the eye, or a foreign object is embedded in it:

· do not attempt to examine the eye;

· do not allow the casualty to touch the eye;

· do not attempt to remove a foreign object that is embedded in the eye;

· call for medical assistance.

1 While you are waiting for medical assistance to arrive, reassure the casualty and then lay him or her down, if possible, or seated comfortably.

2 With the casualty lying on his or her back or seated comfortably, place a light dressing (see pages 68 to 72) over both eyes, making sure that there is no pressure on the injured eye's lid. If necessary, place some additional padding above, and below, the eyelid before lightly placing the dressing over the top. Ask the casualty not to move his or her eyes.

2

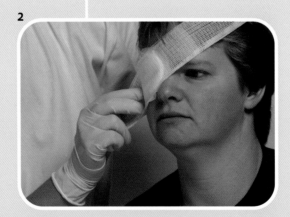

Treating smoke in the eyes

A casualty who has been in a fire may have smoke in his or her eyes, and may therefore have closed them tightly. Before doing anything else:
· assess the scene for danger and check the casualty's response (see page 37);
· if necessary, follow the ABC procedure – airway, breathing and circulation (pulse) (see pages 38 to 41);
· call for emergency medical assistance;
· be prepared to resuscitate (see pages 44 to 53) if necessary;
· look for signs of shock (see pages 92 to 94) and be prepared to treat it.

Then ask the casualty not to rub his or her eyes before washing them with a gentle stream of cold water.

Burns to the eyes

Immediate treatment is required for burns to the eyes, which can be caused by heat or chemicals, such as acids and caustic soda, while flash burns can be caused by flashes from an arc-welder.

The signs and symptoms of burns to the eyes

The signs and symptoms of burns to the eyes include:
· pain in the eyes;
· sensitivity to light;
· severely 'weeping' eyes;
· reddened eyeballs;
· swollen eyelids;
· a possible delayed sensation of 'grit' under the eyelids, especially in the case of flash burns.

Bone, joint and muscle injuries

Treating chemical and heat burns to the eyes

Before treating chemical or heat burns to the eyes:
· assess the scene for danger and check the casualty's response (see page 37);
· if necessary, follow the ABC procedure – airway, breathing and circulation (pulse) (see pages 38 to 41);
· call for emergency medical assistance;
· be prepared to resuscitate (see pages 44 to 53) if necessary;
· look for signs of shock (see pages 92 to 94) and be prepared to treat it.

Then take the following steps.
1 Gently open the casualty's eye with your fingers and then flush it with a gentle stream of cool water for at least twenty minutes.
2 Apply a light, sterile dressing (see page 71) or eye pad and then seek medical assistance as a matter of urgency.

Treating flash burns to the eyes

To treat flash burns to the eyes, follow the first-aid procedure outlined above for treating chemical and heat burns, but omit step 1, that is, do not flush the eye with water before applying a sterile dressing and seeking medical assistance.

1
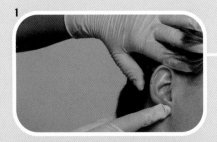

2
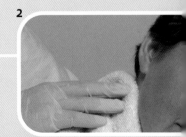

Ear injuries

The ear is prone to several types of injury. The outer part of the ear and the lobe bleed copiously when injured, and the bleeding is best controlled by applying pressure for ten minutes with a dressing or pad made of a clean, non-fluffy material, such as a folded handkerchief, after which medical attention should be sought. Bleeding from inside the ear canal can be the result of a scratch or infected spot within the ear. More seriously, however, it can also be caused by a blow or explosive blast, which may rupture the eardrum. A blow to the head that has fractured the skull may also cause bleeding from the ear.

Managing small foreign objects in the ear

Small objects, such as grass seeds and insects, can enter the ear, and young children often insert beads and matchsticks, for example, into their ears. Foreign bodies in the ear may cause temporary deafness, may damage the eardrum and, if left untreated, may cause infection.

If you think that a foreign object has entered the casualty's ear:

· do not probe inside the ear, but instead look into it to try to identify the object and see how deeply it is positioned;

· do not attempt to remove any foreign object (unless it is an insect, in which case follow the steps below), but instead take the casualty to hospital.

To remove an insect from the casualty's ear, do the following.

1 Reassure the casualty and ask him or her to tilt the head to one side, so that the affected ear is uppermost. Place a towel over that shoulder and support the head with your hand.

2 Using a pipette or the corner of a handkerchief, drop one droplet of very slightly warmed vegetable oil (or else a little tepid water) into the casualty's affected ear. The insect should float to the surface of the ear. If it does not, however, take the casualty to hospital.

Bone, joint and muscle injuries

Managing bleeding from the ear

Bleeding from the ear may be a symptom of a perforated eardrum (see below), a fractured skull or other type of serious injury caused by either a blow to the head or a fall. Before managing a case of bleeding from the ear:

· assess the scene for danger and check the casualty's response (see page 37);

· if necessary, follow the ABC procedure – airway, breathing and circulation (pulse) (see pages 38 to 41);

· call for emergency medical assistance;

· be prepared to resuscitate (see pages 44 to 53) if necessary;

· look for signs of shock (see pages 92 to 94) and be prepared to treat it.

The next steps are as follows.

1 Reassure the casualty and then, even if he or she is conscious, place him or her in the recovery position (see pages 42 to 43), so that the affected ear is facing downwards, towards the ground.

2 Place a sterile pad, or a pad made of a clean, non-fluffy material, such as a folded handkerchief, between the casualty's ear and the ground. Allow the blood to drain away freely and seek medical assistance as a matter of urgency. Remember:

· do not plug the ear canal;

· do not administer eardrops of any kind;

· allow the blood or fluid to drain away freely from the ear;

· seek medical assistance urgently.

A perforated eardrum

The eardrum is a sensitive membrane that lies across the passage between the middle and inner ears. It may be perforated (or ruptured) by pressure changes during flying or scuba-diving, by a blow to the head, an explosion, an infection or a foreign object. Essential for hearing, damage to the eardrum can result in deafness.

The signs and symptoms of a perforated eardrum

The signs and symptoms of a perforated eardrum include:
· severe pain in the affected ear;
· no, or reduced, hearing in the affected ear;
· blood or fluid escaping from inside the ear.

Managing a perforated eardrum

Before managing a perforated eardrum:
· assess the scene for danger and check the casualty's response (see page 37);
· if necessary, follow the ABC procedure – airway, breathing and circulation (pulse) (see pages 38 to 41);
· call for emergency medical assistance;
· be prepared to resuscitate (see pages 44 to 53) if necessary;
· look for signs of shock (see pages 92 to 94) and be prepared to treat it.
 Thereafter, do the following.
1 Reassure the casualty and place him or her in the recovery position (see pages 42 o 43), so that the affected ear is facing downwards, towards the ground.
2 Place a sterile pad, or a pad made of a clean, non-fluffy material, such as a folded handkerchief, between the casualty's ear and the ground. Allow the blood to drain away freely and immediately seek medical assistance. Remember:
· do not plug the ear canal;
· do not administer eardrops of any kind;
· allow the blood or fluid to drain away freely from the ear;
· seek medical assistance urgently.

Bone, joint and muscle injuries

Nose injuries

The nose contains many blood vessels, which lie close to the surface of the nostrils' inner lining. If these blood vessels are injured – perhaps by a knock or blow to the outside of the nose or head, by blowing or sneezing the nose too hard or by picking and poking around inside the nostrils – the common nosebleed may be the result.

Managing a nosebleed

Although the everyday nosebleed is seldom serious, any persistent bleeding may indicate a more serious injury, and medical attention should therefore be sought.

When treating a nosebleed, take the following steps.

1 Tell the casualty not to blow his or her nose and to breathe through the mouth. Place cold, wet towels on the forehead and neck to keep the casualty cool. As soon as possible, sit the casualty down, with the head inclined slightly forwards, and pinch the nostrils immediately below the nasal bone with your forefinger and thumb. Tell the casualty not to move his or her head while you maintain this pressure for at least ten minutes.

2 After ten minutes, release the pressure very gradually (the casualty's head should still be held forwards) and then wipe around the nose and mouth with a sterile swab or a dressing soaked in lukewarm water. Advise the casualty not to blow his or her nose for at least four hours.

If the bleeding persists, repeat steps 1 and 2.

If the blood then still continues to flow, ask the casualty to hold his or her own nose and maintai the pressure as outlined in step 1. Now seek medical assistance.

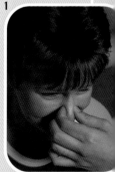

1

Managing a foreign object in the nostril

Young children commonly insert foreign objects such as beans, peas, marbles, crayons and buttons into their nostrils. If this happens, even if you can see it clearly, do not try to remove it with either your fingers or an instrument, such as tweezers, because there is a danger that you could push or lodge it further up the nose, where it could block the airway.

Instead, if the object is small, tell the casualty to breathe through his or her mouth and to block the opposite nostril with a finger. Now tell the casualty to blow through his or her nose, which may blow the object out.

If this fails, however, tell the casualty to resume breathing through his or her mouth while you seek medical treatment as a matter of urgency.

Treating a broken nose or cheekbone

A forceful blow may fracture the nose or cheekbone, causing painful swelling that may block the casualty's airway. Although there may also be bleeding, unless it is severe, do not apply any pressure to the injury because this will cause more pain. Be alert for signs of shock (see pages 92 to 94) and for the casualty's airway (see page 38) being blocked by swelling.

Treat a broken nose or cheekbone by placing a cold compress (see page 127) on the injured area to reduce the swelling and pain. If the bleeding is severe, treat it as you would a nosebleed (see page 166) and then seek medical attention.

If a clear, yellowish fluid is leaking from the nose, assume that the casualty has a skull fracture, treat it accordingly (see page 156) and call for emergency assistance.

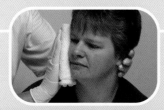

Bone, joint and muscle injuries

Injuries to the mouth and tongue

Injuries inside the mouth are often self-inflicted, being caused by accidentally biting the inside of the cheeks or lips. Although the resultant bleeding can be quite copious, it can quickly be stopped by covering the wound with a clean dressing, firmly pinching the injured area between the forefinger and thumb and applying gentle pressure to both sides. If, however, the bleeding does not stop within two to three minutes, seek medical attention.

To stop a bitten tongue from bleeding, stick it out and then grasp it firmly, but gently, with a clean cloth. This constricts the blood vessels at the base of the tongue and should stop the bleeding within ten minutes. If the bleeding persists, however, seek medical attention.

Injuries to the gums

Bleeding from the gums is usually triggered by brushing one's teeth and nearly always indicates gum disease, although it can also be the result of an incorrect, or overly hard and vigorous, brushing technique. Bleeding from the gums is seldom serious, but a visit to the dentist is nevertheless strongly advised.

Treating a bleeding tooth socket

A tooth socket will bleed following a tooth extraction, the accidental loss or dislodgement of a tooth or after the jaw has been fractured (see page 171).

To stem the bleeding, first tell the casualty not to poke the socket with his or her tongue. Then place a firm gauze pad (thick enough to prevent the top and bottom teeth from meeting) over the socket and ask the casualty to bite on the pad for ten to twenty minutes. After the bleeding has stopped, advise the casualty not to drink anything hot for twelve hours and not to poke the clot with his or her tongue or to try to rinse it away.

If the socket bleeds for more than thirty minutes, replace the gauze pad with a fresh one and then seek medical or dental advice.

Treating an adult whose tooth has been knocked out

If the casualty's tooth has been knocked out, replace it in its socket, making sure that you don't handle the root and that you've positioned it the right way round. Hold it in place for two minutes and then mould a piece of gauze over it and the tooth on each side of it to act as a splint. Place a gauze pad between the top and bottom teeth to keep the 'splint' in position and then take the casualty to a dentist.

If the casualty can't cope with the above procedure, he or she could hold the knocked-out tooth inside the mouth, against the cheek. Alternatively, place it in a glass or cup and cover it with milk or water – or, better still, the casualty's saliva – before seeking emergency dental treatment.

Bone, joint and muscle injuries

A dislocated jaw

Dislocations of any joint – the knees, hips or shoulders, for example – can occur when the bones that form their joins are forced into an abnormal relationship. A jaw can sometimes be dislocated simply by yawning too widely!

The signs and symptoms of a dislocated jaw

The signs and symptoms of a dislocated jaw include:
· an inability to close the mouth;
· drooling;
· pain in front of the ear;
· tenderness.

Managing a dislocated jaw

The procedure for managing a dislocated jaw is as follows:
· do not attempt to move or 'click' the joint back into position because this could damage the surrounding nerves and tissues and worsen a fracture;
· do not give the casualty anything to eat or drink;
· remove any dentures;
· support the lower jaw in the position that is the most comfortable for the casualty;
· seek medical aid.

A fractured jaw

A fractured jaw is usually the result of a direct blow. Note that a blow to one side of the jaw can cause a fracture on the other side.

The signs and symptoms of a fractured jaw

The signs and symptoms of a fractured jaw include:
· severe pain;
· an inability to chew;
· tenderness and swelling;
· deformity or misalignment of the jaw and teeth;
· drooling.

Managing a fractured jaw

Before managing a fractured jaw, do the following:
· assess the scene for danger and check the casualty's response (see page 37);
· if necessary, follow the ABC procedure – airway, breathing and circulation (pulse) (see pages 38 to 41);
· call for emergency medical assistance;
· be prepared to resuscitate (see pages 44 to 53) if necessary;
· look for signs of shock (see pages 92 to 94) and be prepared to treat it.
  If the casualty is unconscious, place him or her in the recovery position (see pages 42 to 43).
If the casualty is conscious (and other injuries permit it), place him or her in the position that is the most comfortable, which is usually sitting up and leaning forwards.
  In both cases, either support the jaw with your hand or gently pull the lower jaw forwards to keep the airway open (see page 38); if the casualty is conscious, he or she may be able to support the injured jaw. Then seek medical assistance as a matter of urgency.

Bone, joint and muscle injuries

Chest injuries

Chest injuries can range from minor contusions (bruises) that are evident on the skin to more serious injuries that may affect the casualty's breathing and circulation and cause life-threatening damage to his or her vital organs. These types of injury include:

· fractured ribs;
· flail chest;
· penetrating chest wounds, such as stab and bullet wounds;
· such lung injuries as bruising, bleeding, collapse and the leakage of air or blood into the chest cavity.

Fractured ribs

Fractured ribs may either be closed fractures (see page 134) or the ribs may have been forced into, and have damaged, the lungs. As a result, blood and air may be escaping into the chest cavity. If a chest injury damages several ribs, the casualty's breathing may be badly affected.

The signs and symptoms of fractured ribs

The signs and symptoms of fractured ribs include:
· pain, which increases as the casualty breathes and coughs;
· difficulty in breathing, and the casualty's breathing pattern may be short, rapid and gasping;
· the casualty supporting the injured side of the chest with an arm or hand;
· tenderness at the injury site;
· frothy, bloodstained sputum;
· possibly a crackling sound.

Managing fractured ribs

The management of a casualty with fractured ribs depends on whether he or she is conscious.

If the casualty is conscious, look for, and be prepared to treat, signs of shock (see pages 92 to 94). Thereafter, take the following steps.

1 Place the casualty in a comfortable position (other injuries permitting), which is usually half-sitting and leaning in the direction of the injured side. Ask the casualty to breathe with short breaths, using his or her diaphragm. Gently position ample padding over the injured area.

2 Apply one or two broad bandages (see page 83), securing the affected arm and padding to the injured side of the chest and tying the bandages with a reef knot (see page 73) on the uninjured side. If the bandages increase the casualty's pain or discomfort, remove them.

3 Immobilise the arm with either a collar-and-cuff or elevation (St John) sling (see pages 88 and 89) and then seek medical assistance as a matter of urgency.

If the casualty is unconscious:

· assess the scene for danger and check the casualty's response (see page 37);

· if necessary, follow the ABC procedure – airway, breathing and circulation (pulse) (see pages 38 to 41);

· be prepared to resuscitate (see pages 44 to 53) if necessary;

· look for signs of shock (see pages 92 to 94) and be prepared to treat it.

. control any bleeding (see pages 95 to 105);

· lay the casualty on his or her uninjured side and seek medical assistance urgently.

Bone, joint and muscle injuries

Flail chest

When several ribs have been broken, and in more than one place, the affected part of the ribcage becomes loose and doesn't move with the rest of the ribcage when the casualty breathes, instead moving in the opposite direction. This is called 'paradoxical breathing'.

The signs and symptoms of flail chest

The signs and symptoms of flail chest include:
· gasping for air;
· severe chest pain;
· difficulty breathing and speaking;
· blue lips
· paradoxical breathing;
· possible unconsciousness.

Managing flail chest

Before managing a case of flail chest:

· assess the scene for danger and check the casualty's response (see page 37);

· if necessary, follow the ABC procedure – airway, breathing and circulation (pulse) (see pages 38 to 41);

· call for emergency medical assistance;

· be prepared to resuscitate (see pages 44 to 53) if necessary;

· control any bleeding (see pages 95 to 105);

· look for signs of shock (see pages 92 to 94) and be prepared to treat it.

After that, take the following steps.

1 Place the casualty in as comfortable a position as possible, usually half-sitting and leaning in the direction of the injured side. If the casualty is unconscious, however, place him or her in the recovery position (see pages 42 to 43).

2 Loosen any tight clothing and then position a large, bulky dressing over the affected area and firmly secure it with a bandage (see pages 68 to 72).

3 Bend the arm on the injured side at the elbow and ensure that the fingers of that hand are pointing towards the opposite shoulder. Now securely bandage the arm to the chest and wait for medical assistance to arrive.

Penetrating chest wounds

A puncture or stab wound can leave a deceptively small hole in the skin. The wound underneath may be large, however, and a deep wound to the chest may puncture a lung, causing air to be sucked into, and out of, the chest cavity, the lung to collapse and blood to accumulate between the lung and the chest wall.

Bone, joint and muscle injuries

The signs and symptoms of a penetrating chest wound

The signs and symptoms of a penetrating chest wound include:
· pain at the site of the injury;
· shortness of breath;
· a visible wound or blood-stained clothing;
· a sucking noise coming from the wound;
· possible unconsciousness.

Managing a penetrating chest wound

Before managing a penetrating chest wound:
· assess the scene for danger and check the casualty's response (see page 37);
· if necessary, follow the ABC procedure – airway, breathing and circulation (pulse) (see pages 38 to 41);
· call for emergency medical assistance as a matter of urgency;
· be prepared to resuscitate (see pages 44 to 53) if necessary;
· look for signs of shock (see pages 92 to 94) and be prepared to treat it.
Then do the following.
1 If the casualty is conscious, place him or her in the most comfortable position, usually half-sitting and leaning in the direction of the injured side. If the casualty is unconscious, place him or her in the recovery position (see pages 42 to 43).
2 Ask someone to bring you an airtight dressing, such as a plastic sheet, a plastic bag or some kitchen foil, and some adhesive tape and place your hand over the wound until they arrive. Then tape the top edge and both sides, but not the bottom edge, of the airtight dressing to the wound with adhesive tape and wait for the emergency services to arrive. If an airtight dressing and adhesive tape are not available, cover the wound with a sterile dressing or pad made of a piece of clean, non-fluffy material.
3 If the casualty's breathing becomes more difficult, remove the dressing or pad.

Abdominal and pelvic injuries

If such organs as the liver, pancreas or spleen have been damaged by an injury to the abdominal area, severe internal bleeding may result, while an injury to the bowels can result in the contents of the intestines spilling into the abdominal cavity, causing inflammation and infection. A major feature of abdominal injuries is shock (see pages 92 to 94).

Injuries to the pelvis are often the result of motor accidents, especially when pedestrians are knocked down by cars, or of being crushed. In both instances, there may be fractures of the pelvis that may also cause damage to the organs located in the pelvic region, namely the bladder and reproductive organs.

The signs and symptoms of an abdominal or pelvic injury

The signs and symptoms of an abdominal or pelvic injury include:
· pain;
· nausea or vomiting;
· difficulty breathing and grunting;
· visible evidence of the injury, such as a wound, bruising, swelling or tenderness;
· rigidity of the abdominal muscles and their resistance to light pressure;
· if the bladder has been injured, blood in the urine;
· if the anus or genitals have been injured, bleeding from these parts of the body;
· in the case of a penetrating abdominal wound, the intestines protruding through the wound;
· an inability to stand;
· shock.

Bone, joint and muscle injuries

Managing an abdominal injury

Before managing an abdominal injury:
· assess the scene for danger and check the casualty's response (see page 37);
· if necessary, follow the ABC procedure – airway, breathing and circulation (pulse) (see pages 38 to 41);
· call for emergency medical assistance;
· be prepared to resuscitate (see pages 44 to 53) if necessary;
· look for signs of shock (see pages 92 to 94) and be prepared to treat it.

Then take the following steps.

1 Loosen the casualty's clothing. Do not give him or her anything to eat or drink, although you can moisten the casualty's lips if he or she is thirsty. Position the casualty on his or her back, with the head and shoulders slightly raised and the knees supported by rolled-up blankets or clothes.

2 If the intestines are protruding through the wound, cover them with a large, non-adhesive, sterile dressing, such as kitchen foil or clingfilm, preferably soaked in sterile saline solution or clean water. Now wait for medical assistance to arrive.

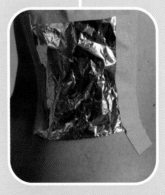

Managing a pelvic injury

Before managing a pelvic injury:
· assess the scene for danger and check the casualty's response (see page 37);
· if necessary, follow the ABC procedure – airway, breathing and circulation (pulse) (see pages 38 to 41);
· call for emergency medical assistance;
· be prepared to resuscitate (see pages 44 to 53) if necessary;
· look for signs of shock (see pages 92 to 94) and be prepared to treat it.

1 If the casualty is conscious, position him or her flat on the back, with the knees slightly bent and supported by rolled-up blankets or clothes.
2 If applicable, remove the contents of the casualty's hip pockets and reassure him or her. The casualty may have a strong urge to urinate, and if this happens, offer further reassurance. Now wait for medical assistance to arrive.

Managing a casualty who has swallowed a foreign object

Although young children are especially prone to putting objects in their mouths and accidentally swallowing them, adults do this, too: remember how many times you've held nails, screws, pins, pen tops and other assorted odds and ends in your mouth to free up both hands!

If this happens, do not allow the casualty to eat or drink anything and seek medical attention immediately.

Bone, joint and muscle injuries

Chapter 6

Acute illness

Many people live their daily lives dealing with conditions that must be controlled with medication, such as asthma, diabetes and epilepsy. Sometimes, however, sufferers may experience sudden attacks of illness, which may cause great discomfort and distress and may, in some instances, even prove fatal without prompt medical attention.

Asthma attacks

Asthma is one of the most common chronic childhood diseases. Once diagnosed, it is controlled with medication, usually in the form of a metered-dose bronchial-dilator aerosol, commonly known as a 'puffer' (very young children may need to use other devices, however). Asthmatics also help to control their condition by ensuring that their homes are as dust-free as possible and by performing special breathing exercises that help to clear the air from the lungs and strengthen the muscles that are used in breathing.

Many asthmatics nevertheless experience attacks in which their breathing becomes seriously restricted by the contraction of the 'air tubes' in the lungs, when the muscles surrounding them go into spasm, the lining of the airways become swollen and excessive mucus is produced. All of these make the tubes narrower, making it difficult to breathe.

Asthma attacks can be caused by allergies, but experiencing emotional or physical stress may also result in an attack. Because most asthma sufferers carry their own medication, they are often able to relieve their breathing difficulties very quickly. A first attack experienced by a child, or a severe attack experienced by a diagnosed sufferer, can be more serious, however, especially if none of the necessary drugs are available or the casualty needs help in locating and administering his or her emergency treatment.

The signs and symptoms of an asthma attack

The signs and symptoms of an asthma attack include:
· difficulty breathing, especially breathing out;
· quiet-sounding breathing during a severe attack;
· rapid, shallow breaths;
· possibly a noisy or wheezing cough;
· tightness across the chest;
· difficulty speaking or moving during a severe attack;
· blueness of the lips;
· confusion;
· tiredness;
· anxiety;
· possible loss of consciousness.

The severity of an asthma attack is difficult to assess, not least because the signs and symptoms vary from person to person. Asthma can occasionally be fatal, which means that prompt action is always required.

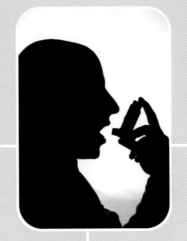

Managing an asthma attack

Ambulances carry equipment with which to deal with asthmatics of all ages, so if the sufferer is not carrying medication, medical assistance should be sought immediately.

When someone suffers an asthma attack:

· do not ask the casualty questions that encourage him or her to talk because this may increase the breathlessness;

· do not force the casualty to lie down during an attack because this may make breathing more difficult.

If the casualty is unconscious, follow the ABC procedure – airway, breathing and circulation (pulse) (see pages 38 to 41) – and then immediately seek medical assistance.

If the casualty is conscious, take the following steps.

1 Reassure the casualty, help him or her to sit down in a comfortable position, preferably in a quiet, airy place, away from other people, and loosen any tight clothing. Assist the casualty to administer his or her medication using the inhaler.

2 Watching the casualty carefully, now wait for ten minutes. In most cases, the dose of medication will have relieved the casualty's breathing difficulties. If, however, the symptoms appear to be getting steadily worse after ten minutes, call for immediate medical assistance. Continue to help the casualty to administer medication from the inhaler (it is very unlikely that he or she will overdose on it).

Acute illness

Diabetes mellitus

Diabetes mellitus is a disorder whereby the body is unable to metabolise glucose (sugar) properly. The body's blood-sugar level is normally regulated by the hormone insulin, which is secreted by the pancreas. Diabetics, however, have to supplement and control their insulin level with either regular insulin injections or orally administered drugs.

Although most diabetics are aware of the dangers inherent in their condition and can avoid them, some wear an identifying 'medic-alert' bracelet or locket or carry a card in their wallet or purse to indicate their illness in case of emergency.

Two serious conditions can affect diabetics: hypoglycaemia and hyperglycaemia.

Hypoglycaemia

Hypoglycaemia occurs when too high a level of insulin causes a low blood-sugar level. Although most diabetics will recognise the onset of an attack, they may need help.

The signs and symptoms of hypoglycaemia

The signs and symptoms of hypoglycaemia include:
· weakness and faintness;
· hunger;
· a pale, sweaty skin;
· a strong pulse and heart palpitations;
· shallow breathing;
· a tingling around the mouth;
· slurred speech;
· confusion and possibly aggressive behaviour;
· possible unconsciousness.

A 'medic-alert' bracelet, locket or card in the casualty's purse or wallet may confirm that he or she has diabetes and may therefore be suffering from hypoglycaemia.

Managing hypoglycaemia

How an attack of hypoglycaemia is managed depends on whether the casualty is conscious or unconscious.

If the casualty is unconscious:
· place him or her in the recovery position (see pages 42 to 43);
· check the ABC: airway, breathing and circulation (pulse) (see pages 38 to 41);
· do not give the casualty anything by mouth;
· seek medical assistance as a matter of urgency.

If the casualty is conscious, take the following steps.

1 Give the casualty some glucose, in the form of lemonade, orange juice, sweet tea or a glass of water with two teaspoons of sugar dissolved in it.

2 Once the casualty is feeling better (which will usually be a few minutes later), give him or her some more complex carbohydrates, such as a sandwich, or even a piece of fruit.

3 Having allowed the casualty to rest for a while, recommend a visit to his or her doctor for advice on how to avoid similar hypoglycaemic attacks in the future.

Acute illness

Hyperglycaemia

Too little insulin can lead to high blood-sugar levels in diabetics. Hyperglycaemia, as it is called, is a dangerous condition that may result in unconsciousness and ultimately a coma.

The signs and symptoms of hyperglycaemia

The signs and symptoms of hyperglycaemia include:
· extreme thirst;
· the need to urinate frequently;
· tiredness or sleepiness;
· a dry, flushed skin;
· a rapid pulse;
· heavy, deep breathing;
· breath that smells of acetone (nail-varnish remover);
· blurred vision;
· nausea, vomiting or abdominal pain;
· possible unconsciousness.

Managing hyperglycaemia

If you suspect that the casualty has hyperglycaemia, call an ambulance immediately.
  If the casualty is unconscious:
· place him or her in the recovery position (see pages 42 to 43);
· check the ABC: airway, breathing and circulation (pulse) (see pages 38 to 41);
· be prepared to resuscitate (see pages 44 to 53) if necessary;
· do not give the casualty anything by mouth.
If the casualty is conscious:
· encourage the casualty to administer insulin him- or herself – do not do this yourself;
· if medical assistance is delayed, encourage the casualty to drink a sugar-free liquid.

Epilepsy

Epilepsy is caused by the disturbance of electrical activity within the brain, causing epileptics to suffer fits. Epileptic fits may be sudden and dramatic, but can sometimes pass unnoticed because the casualty simply appears to be daydreaming. This is because there are two main types of fit: minor fits and major, tonic or clonic fits.

Most people who suffer from epilepsy carry a card or 'medic-alert' bracelet or locket stating so. It is important that you do not become frightened or distressed if you see someone having a major fit; the best way of dealing with the casualty is to understand the nature of the condition and to be able to offer practical help.

Minor fits

Minor fits, sometimes also called petit mal, occur most frequently in children and are rare after the age of thirty. The usual form is characterised by:
· transient lapses in consciousness lasting from five to thirty seconds, with no convulsive seizures;
· a rhythmical, three-per-second blinking of the eyes.

This type of 'absence' seizure may be very mild (occurring less than once a day), and can pass unnoticed (indeed, the condition may go unnoticed for years). Once the condition has been diagnosed, it can be successfully controlled with medication.

Acute illness

Major, tonic or clonic fits

Major, tonic or clonic fits, sometimes also called grand mal, can occur at any age. The length of time between single attacks can vary between several hours and several years.

The signs and symptoms of a major, tonic or clonic fit

The signs and symptoms of a major, tonic or clonic fit include:

· a cry as air is forced through the vocal cords;

· the casualty falling to the ground (which may cause an injury) and lying rigid for a few seconds with the back arched and the jaws clenched;

· a congested, blue face and neck;

· jerking, spasmodic muscle movements and improved colour as normal breathing resumes;

· froth emanating from the mouth, which may sometimes be bloodstained due to the tongue or inside cheek having accidentally been bitten;

· possible loss of bladder or bowel control;

· confusion and a lack of awareness of what has happened for several minutes after the casualty has regained consciousness;

· exhaustion and a tendency to sleep deeply following a fit.

Managing a major fit

The main aims of first aid when someone is suffering a major fit are, firstly, to protect the casualty from injury, but without restricting his or her movement and, secondly, to reassure the casualty when the seizure has passed. Remember that you should:

· never try to hold someone down or stop the convulsions;

· never put anything in the casualty's mouth, including food or drink, during a seizure.

If you are confronted by someone who is having a major fit, do the following.

1 If you can, try to ease the casualty's fall to prevent him or her from being injured. Keep calm and stop onlookers from rushing towards the casualty, and instead clear a space around him or her. If possible, place some padding under, or around, the head. At this stage there is little more that you can do, so let the seizure run its course.

2 When the seizure has abated, loosen any tight clothing, talking reassuringly to the casualty as you do so because a semi-conscious person is easily scared.

3 When the casualty's jerking movements have stopped, check – and, if necessary, open – his or her airway (see page 38), monitor the breathing (see pages 39 to 40) and then place the casualty in the recovery position (see pages 42 to 43).

4 Remain with the casualty when the attack is over and reassure him or her that there has been a complete recovery. If the casualty falls asleep, do not disturb him or her, but check the ABC: airway, breathing and circulation (see pages 38 to 41).

Call for emergency medical assistance in the following instances:

· if a seizure continues for more than five minutes; or

· if the casualty is unconscious for more than ten minutes; or

· if the casualty does not regain consciousness between fits; or

· if this is the casualty's first seizure; or

· if there is a rapidly recurring series of major seizures (*status epilepticus*), which is exhausting for the casualty and may even be fatal.

Acute illness

Febrile convulsions

Babies and children between the ages of six months and six years can suffer from seizures known as febrile convulsions. These are caused by a rise in body temperature (fever) as a result of an infection, which may – or may not – be obvious, fright or a temper tantrum. Although febrile convulsions may look alarming, they are usually not dangerous, and if they are without complications, do not cause any damage or result in epilepsy.

The signs and symptoms of febrile convulsions

The signs and symptoms of febrile convulsions include:
· a flushed or sweating face and a hot forehead;
· the eyes rolling upwards;
· the child holding its breath, resulting in a bluish tinge to the face;
· the back stiffening and arching, followed by the body becoming limp;
· possible unconsciousness.

Managing febrile convulsions

If a child has febrile convulsions, follow the procedure outlined below.

1 During the seizure, place the child in the recovery position (see pages 42 to 43) and keep the airway clear (see page 38). Do not forcibly restrain him or her. If possible, protect the child from injury by removing any potentially dangerous objects nearby.

2 Remove the child's clothing (and if he or she is in bed, any bedclothes) to prevent a further rise in body temperature and clear the space immediately around the child. Wipe away any froth from the mouth.

3 Sponge the child's body with tepid water to reduce the fever, working from the head downwards. Fan the body to assist the cooling process, but do not cool the child too much. (You could also give him or her a proprietary fever-reducing medicine, but before doing so read the instructions on the label to determine the correct dosage.)

4 If possible, keep the child lying on his or her side and cover him or her lightly once the body temperature has come down. Seek medical aid if the child's temperature rises again. It is possible.

If he or she loses consciousness briefly, keep the child in the recovery position while you seek medical attention.

Acute illness

Stroke

A stroke is caused by either the bleeding or blockage (thrombosis) of a blood vessel in the brain, which can result in a wide variety of symptoms, depending on the severity of the stroke and the extent of the damage to the brain. Although strokes are common among elderly people, they can occur in anyone of any age.

The signs and symptoms of a stroke

The signs and symptoms of a stroke include:

· a severe headache, which usually comes on suddenly;
· impaired mobility, ranging from a complete loss of movement and feeling in the arm or leg on one side of the body, which is serious, to clumsiness or perhaps a drooping eyelid, which are minor;
· difficulty swallowing;
· slurred or garbled speech, indicating an altered level of consciousness;
· a pounding pulse;
· the possible turning of the head and eyes to one side;
· a flushed face;
· different-sized pupils;
· possibly seizures.

Managing a stroke

All stroke casualties, regardless of the stroke's degree of severity, require immediate medical attention.

In addition, because they may still be able to hear and understand you, even if they cannot communicate, all stroke casualties need to be constantly reassured.

The procedure for managing a stroke victim who is conscious varies slightly from the first aid required for one who is unconscious.

If the casualty is conscious, do the following.

1 Support the casualty's head and shoulders as you lay him or her down. Put pillows under the head and shoulders to keep them slightly raised and then tilt the head to one side.

2 Loosen any tight clothing, all the while telling the casualty what you are doing.

3 Wipe away any drool from the mouth.

4 Keep the airway clear and open (see page 38). Now seek medical assistance.

If the casualty is unconscious, take the following steps.

1 Follow the ABC procedure – open the casualty's airway, check the breathing and then the circulation (pulse) (see pages 38 too 41) – and be prepared to resuscitate (see pages 44 to 53) if necessary.

2 Seek medical assistance as a matter of urgency.

3 Place the casualty in the recovery position (see pages 42 to 43). Check the ABC at regular intervals while waiting for medical assistance to arrive.

Hysteria

Hysteria is caused by psychological stress. Although it can resemble an epileptic seizure (see page 187), there is an important distinction: a hysterical casualty will not lose consciousness.

Hysteria should not be regarded as attention-seeking behaviour or dismissed as malingering: it is a genuine psychological reaction to stress and may be completely involuntary.

The signs and symptoms of hysteria

The signs and symptoms of hysteria include:
· strange behaviour, with the casualty perhaps shouting, screaming or waving his or her arms and legs around;
· rolling on the ground, becoming rigid, sometimes holding the breath or even going into a trance-like state (but not losing consciousness or causing injury to him- or herself because the casualty always retains sufficient awareness of what is going on around him or her).

Managing hysteria

Despite what you may have seen in the cinema, do not slap a hysterical person to bring him or her round. Instead, take the following steps.
1 Clear away all onlookers. Be understanding, but firm with the casualty and speak in a no-nonsense tone to try to calm him or her down.
2 If possible, distract the casualty by giving him or her a warm drink.
3 When he or she has calmed down, encourage the casualty to see a doctor in case further treatment is necessary.

If, at any time, you are unsure of the casualty's condition, or if he or she becomes unconscious, place the casualty in the recovery position (see pages 42 to 43) and seek immediate medical assistance.

Injuries caused by extremes of temperature

The temperature of the healthy human body is maintained at about 36 to 37°C (97 to 99°F). We are generally good at adapting to different atmospheric temperatures, putting on extra clothes when it's cold and eating high-energy foods to generate additional body heat, and cooling down when it's hot by casting off layers of clothing, drinking plenty of fluids and sweating.

Overexposure to extremely hot or cold conditions can have serious and damaging effects, however: excessively hot or humid conditions create the risk of succumbing to such heat-related illnesses as heat cramps, heat exhaustion and heat stroke, while overexposure to very cold conditions can result in frostbite and hypothermia.

Overexposure to heat

Probably the most common type of injury caused by overexposure to heat is sunburn. Spending too long in the sun's powerful rays, especially in the middle of the day, can cause the skin to become red, inflamed, swollen and blistered, with the skin eventually drying up and peeling away, while long-term exposure to the sun can result in blotchy skin and even skin cancer.

The first sign of overexposure to the sun is red skin, but by that time the damage has already been done. Prevention is therefore the best possible cure for sunburn, which means rubbing a total sun-block product into your skin, wearing a sun hat and protective clothing and avoiding going out in the sunshine at the hottest times of the day.

Acute illness

Heat-related illnesses

There are three types of heat-related illness:

· heat cramps;
· heat exhaustion; and
· heat stroke.

In most cases, all three are completely preventable as long as you:

· protect yourself from the damaging effects of strong sunlight;
· avoid undertaking physical tasks in hot, humid weather unless you are conditioned to both the task and the environment;
· stop working as soon as you experience heat cramps or heat exhaustion and seek medical attention if the condition persists;
· drink sufficient water to satisfy your thirst and avoid alcohol;
· avoid spending long periods in saunas and steam rooms.

Remember also to protect infants and children by not leaving them in hot cars.

The signs and symptoms of heat cramps

The signs and symptoms of heat cramps include:

· painful muscle cramps in the limbs and abdomen, be it during exercise or at rest;
· nausea or vomiting;
· dizziness, weakness or tiredness;
· a moist, cool skin, although the casualty may complain of feeling hot;
· a headache;
· sweating;
· a rapid pulse and quickened breathing;
· lack of co-ordination;
· confusion and irritability.

The signs and symptoms of heat exhaustion

The signs and symptoms of heat exhaustion include those listed for heat cramps above, although the casualty may also complain of:
· a headache that may have lasted for some hours or days;
· thirst;
· loss of appetite.

Managing heat cramps and heat exhaustion

Manage heat cramps and heat exhaustion as follows.

1 Move the casualty to a cool place through which fresh air is circulating. Lay him or her down, loosen any tight clothing and remove any superfluous clothes. Sponge the casualty with cool water – but do not cool him or her down too much – and encourage him or her to drink plenty of fluids. (Commercial preparations are available to combat heat-related illnesses, but remember that they must be diluted according to the instructions given on their labels.)

2 Apply cold compresses or ice packs (see page 127) to any cramped muscles and ask the casualty to stretch them gently, but do not massage them.

If casualty does not recover or vomits, seek medical assistance immediately.

Acute illness

Heatstroke

Because heat stroke is a dangerous, and potentially fatal, condition, early recognition and treatment is vital. It strikes when the body is unable to cool itself by sweating, perhaps due to an illness or to prolonged exposure to heat and humidity. Although it is most common in tropical areas, it can also occur during hot spells in milder climates, when some people will be more at risk than others. These include:

· infants or children who have been left in cars on hot days;
· athletes, especially amateur enthusiasts (such as 'fun-runners'), who attempt long runs on hot days;
· unfit or overweight workers;
· overweight alcoholics, as well as those who overindulge in alcohol on holiday in hot climates;
· elderly and infirm people.

The signs and symptoms of heat stroke
The signs and symptoms of heat stroke include:
· a rise in body temperature to 40°C (104°F) or more;
· hot, flushed, dry skin;
· a headache;
· dizziness;
· nausea or vomiting;
· a rapid, pounding pulse;
· confusion and irritability;
· a rapid loss of consciousness.

Managing heat stroke

The management of heat stroke varies slightly, depending on whether the casualty is unconscious or conscious.

If the casualty is unconscious:

· place him or her in the recovery position (see pages 42 to 43);

· check the ABC – airway, breathing and circulation (pulse) (see pages 38 to 41) – and be prepared to resuscitate (see pages 44 to 53) if necessary;

· call for emergency medical assistance and then proceed to step 1.

If the casualty is conscious (or breathing spontaneously and the pulse is detectable when the casualty is in the recovery position), do the following.

1 If possible, move the casualty to a cool place. Loosen his or her clothing or, if possible, remove it. Place the casualty in a comfortable position, usually half-lying and half-sitting, with the back and shoulders supported.

2 Cool the casualty as quickly as possible by either applying ice packs, if these are available, to the groin, neck and armpits or wrapping the casualty in a cool, wet sheet and then keeping it wet; alternatively, sponge the casualty's body with cool water. Increase the cooling process by fanning the casualty. Then call for emergency medical assistance.

3 Take the casualty's temperature, which must fall to either:

· 38°C (100.4°F) if taken under the tongue; or

· 37.5°C (99.5°F) if taken under the armpit.

4 Once the casualty's temperature has returned to normal, if you have wrapped him or her in a cool, wet sheet, exchange it for a dry one. Monitor the ABC until medical assistance arrives.

Acute illness

Overexposure to the cold

Overexposure to the cold can occur:
· following immersion in cold water;
· as a result of being exposed to a cold wind;
· if unconscious or immobile casualties are exposed to a cold environment;
· if young children, infants and elderly people are exposed to a cold environment;
· if clothing is inadequate or insufficient for cold weather conditions.

The severity of someone's reaction to being exposed to a cold environment depends on:
· the person's age and physical condition;
· the atmospheric temperature;
· the wind speed;
· the length of exposure.
Aggravating factors furthermore include wind, snow and rain, fatigue, anxiety and hunger.

Frostbite

Frostbite occurs when extreme cold causes the tiny blood vessels in the skin to narrow, thereby cutting off the supply of blood to the extremities, that is, the fingers, toes and nose. If the blood vessels freeze and the blood supply is cut off for a long period, the affected areas may become gangrenous and will then require amputation.

The signs and symptoms of frostbite

The signs and symptoms of frostbite include:
· numbness and tingling in exposed parts of the body;
· skin that suddenly turns white and takes on a waxy appearance;
· firmness of the affected areas to the touch;
· lack of pain in the affected areas;
· the affected areas turning from white to red and becoming swollen; in severe cases, they may turn blue, and then black.

Managing frostbite

As well as seeking medical assistance, the aim of first aid is to warm the frostbitten areas slowly, in order to prevent further tissue damage from occurring, as follows:
· if possible, move the casualty under shelter, to a warm, dry place;
· provide blankets and hot drinks to encourage the casualty to warm up naturally;
· remove any clothing, such as gloves or boots, or jewellery that may be constricting the affected body parts;
· discourage movement and keep the frostbitten areas still;
· cover any blisters with loose, sterile dressings (see pages 68 to 72).

There are certain things that you must not do:
· do not massage the frostbitten areas;
· do not warm the frostbitten areas with hot-water bottles;
· do not thaw a frostbitten foot if the casualty will be required to walk;
· do not apply snow or cold water to the frostbitten areas;
· do not warm the frostbitten areas by applying direct heat;
· do not give the casualty any alcohol to drink.

The next steps are as follows.

1 Either cover the casualty, including the frostbitten parts of the body, with blankets or tuck the casualty's hands under his or her own armpits and place his or her feet under your armpits.

2 Seek medical assistance as a matter of urgency, not least because when the frostbitten parts begin to thaw, they will become extremely painful.

Acute illness

Hypothermia

Hypothermia occurs when the body's temperature drops below the normal 37°C (98.6°F), which may happen if the body's heat-producing mechanism – shivering – ceases to function adequately, perhaps if the body is being constantly cooled by exposure to the wind, for example. Elderly and frail people, especially if they are thin, tired and hungry, are particularly prone to hypothermia, which can strike in homes that are not adequately heated.

The signs and symptoms of hypothermia
The signs and symptoms of hypothermia include:
· initial shivering, which may then abate;
· cold, dry skin;
· a slow pulse;
· slow breathing;
· a below-normal body temperature when measured;
· drowsiness, which may progress to unconsciousness and then cardiac arrest;
· signs of frostbite to the extremities, especially if the casualty has been exposed to extremely cold weather conditions.

Managing hypothermia
The aim of first aid is to warm the body gradually, but without delay, but the treatment varies according to the circumstances, as follows.

If the casualty is conscious and inside, take the following steps.

1 If the casualty has been brought inside in wet clothing, remove his or her clothes and replace them with warm, dry garments as soon as possible.

If the casualty is young and fit, fill a bath with warm water (40°C or 104°F) and help him or her into it.

If the casualty is an infant or an elderly person, wrap him or her in blankets.

2 Once the casualty is in either bed or a warm bath, give him or her warm drinks, such as soup or hot chocolate, and high-energy foods. Because a great amount of body heat is lost from this part of the body, cover the casualty's head (but not the face) with a woolly hat. Now call for medical assistance.

If the casualty is conscious, but outside, proceed as follows.

1 Seek help immediately.

2 Remove any wet clothing and replace it with dry garments.

3 Shelter the casualty by wrapping him or her in a survival bag, blanket or sleeping bag, if necessary sharing your own body heat with the casualty under a common cover.

4 Check the casualty's breathing and circulation (pulse) (see pages 38 to 41).

5 Look for, and if necessary treat, signs of frostbite (see pages 200 to 201).

6 If possible, give the casualty a warm drink, such as milk, cocoa, hot chocolate or soup.

Do not do the following:

· give the casualty a hot-water bottle because this would divert blood from the major organs to the superficial vessels of the skin;

· give the casualty any alcohol to drink;

· rub casualty's limbs or encourage vigorous movement.

7 Reassure and comfort the casualty while waiting for medical assistance to arrive.

If the casualty is unconscious, follow the ABC procedure – check the airway, breathing and circulation (pulse) (see pages 38 to 41) – and be prepared to resuscitate (see pages 44 to 53) if necessary.

If he or she does not show any signs of life, do not assume that the casualty is dead. Because hypothermia protects the brain from the damage caused by lack of oxygen, many hypothermic people survive a period of cardiac arrest (see pages 120 to 121) for longer than is otherwise usual.

Acute illness

Chapter 7

Poisons, bites and stings

Accidental poisoning, caused by swallowing or inhaling poisonous substances can easily be avoided. Most often, the victims are children who explore the cupboards under the sink, where cleaning substances are stored, or garden sheds and garages, where a whole range of toxic substances can be found. Accidental poisoning can be avoided if common-sense precautions are taken regarding the storage of such materials.

Poisons

Poisons can be swallowed, inhaled, injected or absorbed. Many everyday household substances are poisonous, and accidental poisoning can often be prevented by the correct and safe storage of such chemicals.

Two major groups of chemicals cause poisoning when they are swallowed.

1 Poisons that act directly on the mouth, throat, stomach and the rest of the digestive system (although symptoms caused by absorption may occur later). Typical causes of this type of poisoning are contaminated or rotten food and some poisonous plants. Some of these poisons are corrosive, causing immediate damage and pain, and include household bleach, gasoline, strong acids, alkalis like caustic soda (which products like oven cleaners sometimes contain).

2 Poisons that act on the nervous system after they have been absorbed by the body. Because their effects are delayed, and because immediate first aid may not have been given, they are very dangerous. Indeed, when the symptoms appear, severe damage to the body has already been done, and it is usually too late to remove the poison from the system by inducing vomiting. Among these poisons are counted aspirin, paracetamol and other pain-reducing drugs, sleeping tablets and poisonous toadstools.

Other forms of poisoning are caused by inhaling toxic fumes, such as carbon monoxide and fumes from polyurethane foam, or by injections of chemical substances through the skin (by hypodermic syringes or animal or insect bites and stings) or even by splashes to the eye. Finally, certain garden and agricultural chemicals, such as insecticides and organophosphates, can be absorbed through the skin in sufficient quantities to cause poisoning, permanent damage to the body and sometimes even death.

Poisons and poisoning: the rules

Avoid accidental poisoning, protect yourself and treat victims of poisoning by observing the following rules.

· Avoid accidental poisoning by keeping all medicines, household cleaners, DIY solvents and garden chemicals out of children's reach. Never decant chemicals into juice bottles and never replace the childproof tops of bottles and jars deliberately loosely to make them easier to open because this will make it easier for children, too!

· When confronted by a victim of poisoning, take care not to become contaminated yourself, be it by inhaling fumes or coming into contact with liquid chemicals. If you need to administer artificial respiration (AR, see pages 44 to 46), be careful not to transfer any of the poison that the casualty may have swallowed to your own mouth: if possible, wash the casualty's face before administering AR, use the mouth-to-nose method of AR (see page 46) or cut a slit in a plastic bag and cover the casualty's face with the bag before administering breaths through the slit.

· If a casualty has swallowed a corrosive poison, never try to induce vomiting because the poisonous substance that has burnt the casualty's mouth on its way to the stomach will inflict further burns on its way back up again.

· If a casualty does vomit, keep a sample of the vomit to send to hospital with the casualty. This will help to identify the poison, as well as assist emergency staff to calculate how much was ingested.

· Do not try to induce vomiting in an unconscious casualty.

· Do not leave a casualty alone unless you must, in order to call for emergency medical assistance.

The signs and symptoms of poisoning

The signs and symptoms of poisoning include:

· a nearby container containing a poisonous substance;

· unconsciousness, or the loss of consciousness at any time, depending on how much poison has been ingested;

· possible convulsions;

· difficulty breathing;

· an upset stomach, indicated by vomiting (but do not induce vomiting) or diarrhoea;

· damage to the lips and surrounding skin caused by swallowing a corrosive poison: the skin may be burned, blistered or stained yellow, grey or white.

Poisons, bites and stings

The signs and symptoms of poisoning

Before managing a case of poisoning, do the following:
· do not become a casualty yourself, but assess the scene for danger, taking particular note of any chemical spills or toxic fumes;
· check the casualty's ABC – airway, breathing and circulation (pulse) (see pages 38 to 41) – and be prepared to resuscitate (see pages 44 to 53) if necessary;
· immediately call for emergency medical assistance, if possible giving details of the substance involved (the emergency operator will advise you what to do while waiting for the ambulance to arrive).

If the casualty is conscious:
· if the poison is a toxic chemical, such as a pesticide, that can be absorbed through the skin, tell the casualty to remove all contaminated clothes and footwear, to place them in a bag and then to seal it. (If you help the casualty to do this, put on rubber gloves.) Tell the casualty to wash the contaminated parts of his or her skin thoroughly with soap and water;
· do not induce vomiting;
· follow any instructions that the emergency operator has given you;
· when the ambulance arrives, give the crew whatever you think was responsible, be it tablets or a container that you know, or suspect, contained the poisonous substance.

If the casualty is unconscious or loses consciousness:
· place him or her in the recovery position (see pages 42 to 43) before calling for medical assistance as a matter of urgency;
· check the casualty's ABC – airway, breathing and circulation (pulse) (see pages 38 to 41) – and be prepared to resuscitate (see pages 44 to 53) if necessary, remembering to wipe any poisonous substance from the casualty's mouth first.

Bites and stings

Bites and stings can cause great discomfort and distress and sometimes require medical attention. Following an animal bite, for example, a casualty may require stitches, antibiotics or a tetanus injection, or a casualty may suffer a severe allergic reaction to what would, in others, simply be a painful bite or sting, which must be treated immediately.

In many parts of the world, humans co-exist with dangerous species of snake, spider, insect and marine life. Although human contact with such species is generally rare, as their natural habitat is increasingly invaded by land development and tourism, chance encounters are becoming more likely. It is therefore important that travellers take the time to familiarise themselves with any potentially dangerous species, learn to recognise and avoid them and, in an emergency situation, know how to act quickly, sensibly and knowledgeably. (See pages 218 to 239 for a list of dangerous snakes, spiders and marine creatures, along with information on their habitat.)

With climate changes in progress, we should also expect to see the migration of many such species to formerly moderate climates (the normally cool waters around the British Isles, for instance, have already seen increased numbers of weever fish and jellyfish, as well as the arrival in southern counties of larger, and more aggressive, wasps that were formerly confined to continental Europe).

Animal bites

Animal (and human) mouths contain large numbers of organisms, some of which are capable of transmitting serious infections and potentially fatal diseases, such as rabies. Any animal or human bite that punctures or penetrates the skin should therefore be taken seriously.

Following a bite in a part of the world where rabies is present, both the bite victim (who will require hospital treatment) and the suspect animal must undergo medical examination in order to verify or exclude a rabies infection. The culprit animal must therefore be isolated and then caught, but only if it is safe to do so, and if a suspected rabid animal escapes, inform the police or local authorities immediately. Travellers are in any case advised not to approach stray dogs, cats or other animals.

Bites and scratches inflicted by wild animals carry an increased risk of infection, so seek medical advice without delay if you are bitten.

Although the bites and scratches inflicted by domestic cats are not usually deep, they do require cleaning, not least because they often sting. Small pets, such as hamsters, guinea pigs and rabbits, can administer very deep and painful bites, which may need further treatment after the wound has been cleaned and dressed.

Managing a dogbite

Dog bites are usually treated as 'dirty' wounds, and it is important that no more dirt is introduced to the wound while it is being cleaned, as follows.

1 Wipe away any obvious dirt from around the wound, wiping from the wound outwards and using a fresh swab soaked with either soap and water or a mildly antiseptic solution for each wipe.

2 Once the superficial dirt has been removed, clean the bite thoroughly under cold, running water. If the wound is bleeding, allow it to continue because this will wash away the germs.

3 A minor bite can then be covered with an adhesive dressing (see page 69), but not a waterproof one. Apply a sterile gauze dressing to a large or deep bite and then report the bite to a doctor in case stitches or a tetanus injection are required.

1
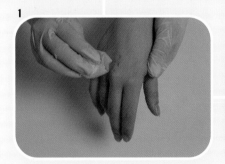

3
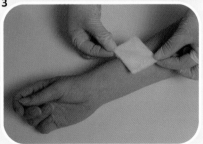

Insect bites

Insect bites are not, in fact, really bites, but are usually the result of a small quantity of material within an insect's saliva, which is injected into the skin by the insect's proboscis, causing an allergic reaction in the form of redness, swelling, itchiness or irritation. This reaction is usually mild, but infection can occur if the wound is scratched and the skin broken. Some reactions can be severe and life-threatening, however, especially if they cause swelling in the larynx (voice box), thus restricting the airway (see page 38).

Bites by mosquitoes and midges may go unnoticed at first because the itching doesn't start until later. Although mosquito bites generally cause nothing more than discomfort, malaria poses a major threat in parts of the world inhabited by the Anopheles mosquito, which transfers parasitic protozoa to the human bloodstream in its bite. If you are travelling to a region where malaria has been identified as being present, seek medical advice well in advance of your departure because you will need to take anti-malarial drugs.

Treating a bee or wasp sting

Not only do bee and wasp stings cause instant pain, but the insect sometimes leaves its sting, which looks like a small splinter, embedded in the skin. Treat a bee or wasp sting as follows.

1 If the sting remains in the skin, remove it with a pair of tweezers, holding them close to the skin to avoid squeezing the sac at the top of the sting and thus forcing more venom into the wound.

2 Wipe the area clean with a sterile swab and apply a cold compress (see page 127).

A sting inside the mouth or throat can be serious because it may cause sufficient swelling to obstruct the airway (see page 38). If you suspect that someone has been stung in the mouth, call for emergency medical assistance and then, if possible, give the casualty an ice cube to suck or a glass of cold water to drink to reduce the swelling.

1

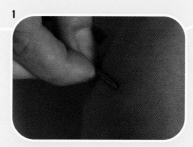

Allergic reactions to insect bites and stings

Some people are extremely sensitive to insect bites and stings (as well as to certain foods, such as nuts), so much so that they may suffer a severe allergic reaction called anaphylactic shock, which can occur very rapidly and cause breathing difficulties. Many such people carry measured-dose medication in the form of adrenaline, which is administered by a syringe called an Epi-pen. Those who do not know that they are sensitive, especially if it is the first time that they have been stung, are especially at risk.

Poisons, bites and stings

The signs and symptoms of anaphylactic shock

The signs and symptoms of anaphylactic shock include:
· local pain, swelling and itching;
· blotchy, red skin;
· puffy eyelids and a swollen face;
· a rapid pulse;
· a constricted throat and breathing difficulties;
· possible unconsciousness.

Treating anaphylactic shock

Treat anaphylactic shock as follows.
1 Help the casualty into a comfortable sitting position to ease any breathing difficulties. If he or she has an Epi-pen, help him or her to administer adrenaline. (Note that if there is any medication that has not been identified by the casualty, a relative or close friend, or the label on the drug, as being required to alleviate an allergic reaction, it must not be administered.) Now seek medical assistance as a matter of urgency.
2 Monitor the casualty's breathing (see pages 39 to 40) and be prepared to administer artificial respiration (see pages 44 to 46) if necessary. If the casualty loses consciousness, place him or her in the recovery position (see page s 42 to 43) and monitor the ABC: airway, breathing and circulation (pulse) (see pages 38 to 41) until the emergency services arrive.

Snakebites

There are more than two-and-a-half-thousand species of snake, most of which are found in the warmer regions of the world. Only a small proportion – about four-hundred species – are venomous and, of those, fewer than a hundred species are dangerous to humans (even in Australia, which has more harmful snakes than harmless ones, fatal bites are rare).

Shy creatures, snakes are not normally aggressive and will only bite when threatened or mishandled. The best advice to avoid being bitten is therefore:

· to leave snakes alone if you come across them in their natural habitat (if you see one, regard yourself as having been fortunate to have experienced a rare sighting);

· to wear sensible, stout shoes when in 'snake country' and not to walk around in sandals or bare feet;

· to make plenty of noise when walking, and to keep your eyes peeled for snakes when moving through long grass;

· not to poke around in piles of wood, rock crevices, the hollows of logs or piles of leaf debris or rubbish because snakes tend to snooze in such places and no one, snakes included, likes to be disturbed when asleep.

In addition, if you share your country or region with snakes:

· don't provide a 'café' for them and instead keep any sheds or outhouses mouse-free;

· keep any grass around your house and children's play areas short;

· use a torch when moving around campsites or farms at night.

The signs and symptoms of a snakebite

Although snakebites cause immediate pain, it is sometimes only later (from between fifteen minutes and two hours) that redness and swelling may appear around the puncture marks. Indeed, there may be no visible signs and symptoms at all. If a person says, or believes, that he or she has been bitten by a snake, however, take him or her seriously.

The signs and symptoms of a snakebite include the following:

· shock (see pages 92 to 94), which is often the greatest risk factor because the casualty may be too shocked to be able to identify the species, and thus whether it is dangerous;

· a headache;
· double vision;
· drowsiness;
· faintness;
· nausea or vomiting and diarrhoea;
· sweating;
· pain or tightness in the chest and abdomen;
· breathing difficulties;
· two puncture marks, or else fang scratches, about 1 cm ($\frac{1}{2}$ in) apart at the site of the bite, which will usually be on a limb, particularly a leg;
· swelling, redness and bruising around the bitten area.

Managing a snakebite

If someone is bitten by a snake, forget what you saw in the cinema and instead follow these rules:

· never cut or excise the bitten area from the casualty's skin;
· never try to suck venom out of the wound;

· never wash the venom off the skin because its traces can help to identify it;
· do not try to catch the snake, although a description of both it and the site of the incident may help to identify its species;
· immediately call for emergency medical assistance.

Before treating the casualty:

· assess the scene for danger;

· check the casualty's ABC: airway, breathing and circulation (pulse) (see pages 38 to 41);

· be alert for, and prepared to treat, the signs of shock (see pages 92 to 94).

Thereafter, take the following steps.

1 Reassure the casualty and then lay him or her down, with the head and shoulders raised and supported, ensuring that the level of the heart is above that of the wound to contain the poison.

2 Wind a wide crêpe or conforming bandage (see pages 74 to 79), or else a piece of clean fabric or even a pair of nylon tights, over the affected area and around the limb, as follows:

· apply the bandage firmly enough to compress the tissues, but not so tightly that it restricts the blood flow;

· bandage from the bite to the fingers or toes, then up to the armpit or groin;

· bandage as much of the limb as possible;

· do not remove the bandage after you have applied it.

3 Support and immobilise the injured limb by either applying a splint (see page 139) with a second bandage or padding it with rolled-up blankets or towels.

4 Check the casualty's breathing and circulation again and be prepared to resuscitate (see pages 44 to 53) if necessary. Also look for, and, if necessary, treat, any signs of shock.

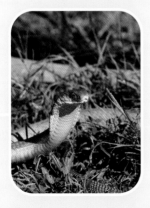

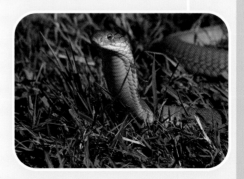

Poisons, bites and stings

This list will help you to identify the dangerous snakes that populate your locality, wherever you are in the world.

Europe

The following dangerous snakes are found in Europe.

Adder
Habitat: heathland, bogs, woods and fields.
Distribution: from north-western Europe, including Britain and Scandinavia, to central and eastern Asia (the largest range of any land snake).
Length: up to 70 cm (27 in).
Colour, markings and features: the males are grey, with a dark-grey or black zigzag down the back; the females are usually brown or a reddish colour, with a dark-brown zigzag; some are plain black; active by day.

Aspic viper
Habitat: dry hillsides and meadows.
Distribution: central Europe and Italy.
Length: up to 60 cm (23 in).
Colour, markings and features: light brown, grey or cream; may have zigzags with a pale centre or a series of dark crossbars down the back joined by a thin, central line; sometimes uniformly black; an upturned snout.

Lataste's viper
Habitat: dry, stony hillsides or sandy areas near the coast (in southern Spain).
Distribution: Spain and Portugal (apart from the northern coasts) and North Africa.
Length: up to 60 cm (23 in).
Colour, markings and features: grey or pale brown, with a wavy zigzag, paler at the centre than at the edges and a row of dark blotches along the sides; a horn on the snout.

Milos viper
Habitat: dry, rocky, scrub-covered valleys and hillsides.
Distribution: the Greek islands of Mílos (Melos), Kimilos, Syphnos and Polyagos.
Length: up to 1 m (3 ft).
Colour, markings and features: usually grey, with faint crossbands of darker grey or orange.

Nose-horned viper
Habitat: dry, rocky places, including dry-stone walls.
Distribution: south-eastern Europe and Turkey.
Length: up to 1 m (3 ft).
Colour, markings and features: silvery-grey, brown or orange, with zigzag markings in a darker shade; a fleshy horn on the tip of the prominent, upturned snout.

North America

The following dangerous snakes are found in North America.

Arizona (or western) coral snake

Habitat: dry places, including the desert, scrub and grassland.

Distribution: southern Arizona and Sonora, Mexico.

Length: about 50 cm (19 in).

Colour, markings and features: patterned with alternate rings of red, white and black, with the red bands bordered on each side by white ones, so that the pattern is black, white, red, white, black and so on.

Banded rock rattlesnake

Habitat: dry, lightly wooded places, scree and among rocks.

Distribution: the southern states of the USA (Texas, New Mexico and Arizona) and north-central Mexico.

Length: about 60 cm (23 in).

Colour, markings and features: usually grey, with dark-brown or grey bands across the body between which are sometimes dark spots; bad-tempered when disturbed, with a warning rattle in the tail.

Black–tailed rattlesnake

Habitat: scrub, semi-desert and lightly wooded areas.

Distribution: south-central USA and central Mexico.

Length: about 1 m (3 ft).

Colour, markings and features: varied colour, from green to yellow, orange or brown; diamonds along the back, although these may be irregular and difficult to distinguish; a distinctive black tail and sometimes a black 'mask' over the face.

Canebrake rattlesnake

Habitat: wooded valleys and thickets.

Distribution: the eastern half of the USA, apart from the Florida peninsula.

Length: 1.3 to 2 m (4 to 6 ft).

Colour, markings and features: brown-grey, with an orange stripe down the centre of the back, interrupted by dark bars or chevrons; the colour becomes darker towards the tail, which may be nearly black; dangerously venomous.

Copperhead

Habitat: rocky hillsides, desert oases and swamps.

Distribution: the south-eastern states of the USA (apart from Florida) and New Mexico.

Length: about 75 cm (29 in).

Colour, markings and features: equal-sized tan, buff or pink bands alternating with dark-red or reddish-brown bands, which may be slightly wider at the sides; the tip of the tail may be yellow.

Cottonmouth

Habitat: swamps, lakes, rivers and ditches.

Distribution: the south-eastern states of the USA.

Poisons, bites and stings

Length: about 1.25 m (4 ft).

Colour, markings and features: brown, dark grey or black, with indistinct crossbands; in Florida especially, a thin, white line passing from the snout to above the eye.

Eastern diamondback rattlesnake

Habitat: pinewoods and scrub.

Distribution: Florida and neighbouring coastal states.

Length: up to 1.7 m (5 ft), but has been recorded at 2.4 m (7 ft), making it the largest rattlesnake in the USA.

Colour, markings and features: brown or olive, with large, dark-brown diamonds along the back, each outlined with light-coloured scales; may have small, dark blotches between the diamonds; two light streaks on the face; produces a warning rattle from the tail if alarmed.

Massassauga

Habitat: damp places, such as swamps and riverbeds.

Distribution: the eastern–central states of the USA (from the Great Lakes to southern Texas) and neighbouring parts of Mexico, but becoming rare.

Length: up to 75 cm (29 in).

Colour, markings and features: dark grey, with dark-brown, elongated blotches along the back; a wide stripe on the snout running to the back of the head; a tiny rattle.

Mojave rattlesnake

Habitat: desert, scrub and rocky areas.

Distribution: the south-western states of the USA and central Mexico.

Length: up to 1 m (3 ft).

Colour, markings and features: grey-green or brown, with oval or diamond marks along the back; may also have a light-coloured stripe running from the eye to the corner of the mouth; banded tail with wide, white and narrow, black rings; very bad-tempered, with extremely potent venom.

Pygmy rattlesnake

Habitat: pinewoods, scrub and swampy places with sandy soil.

Length: up to 50 cm (19 in).

Colour, markings and features: brown, light grey or pinkish in colour; may have a red-orange line down the centre of the back; dark blotches on the back, smaller ones on the sides; a minute rattle, producing a soft, buzzing sound.

Red diamond rattlesnake

Habitat: desert areas.

Distribution: southern California and Baja California, Mexico.

Length: up to 1.5 m (5 ft).

Colour, markings and features: orange, red or reddish-brown in colour, with large, slightly darker diamonds down the back, edged with paler scales; narrow, black-and-white rings in front of the rattle in the tail.

Sidewinder

Habitat: sand dunes or large areas of wind-blown sand.

Distribution: the south-western states of the USA and north-western Mexico.

Length: up to 75 cm (29 in).

Colour, markings and features: the colour may match that of the sand, with a row of darker blotches on the back; horn-like scale above each eye; slender-bodied rattlesnake; moves by side-winding; shuffles under the surface of the sand during the day; is aggressive if disturbed, when it emits a warning rattle.

Texas coral snake

Habitat: dry or moist areas with sandy soil.

Distribution: the south-eastern states of the USA and neighbouring parts of Mexico.

Length: about 75 cm (29 in).

Colour, markings and features: a black snout and wide, yellow band across the head; the rest of the body is marked with wide, red-and-black bands separated by narrow, yellow bands; secretive, tending to hide under logs and tree stumps.

Tiger rattlesnake

Habitat: among cacti on rocky hillsides;

Distribution: southern Arizona and Sonora, Mexico.

Length: about 80 cm (31 in).

Colour, markings and features: grey, pink or mauve, with faint crossbands of a darker shade; a small head, but a large rattle; rarely seen, usually calm, but dangerously venomous.

Timber rattlesnake

Habitat: wooded valleys and thickets.

Distribution: the eastern half of the USA, apart from the Florida peninsula.

Length: 1.3 to 2 m (4 to 6 ft).

Colour, markings and features: yellowish; dangerously venomous.

Western diamondback rattlesnake

Habitat: desert, scrub and grasslands.

Distribution: common in many of the south-western states of the USA, eastern Texas and northern Mexico.

Length: up to 1.7 m (5 ft), but sometimes longer.

Colour, markings and features: may be grey, bluish, pink or black; a series of large, light-edged diamonds down the back and smaller blotches on the snout; two light streaks on the face; wide, black-and-white bands in front of the rattle on the tail.

Western rattlesnake

Habitat: prairies, deserts and foothills.

Distribution: across the western states of the USA into northern Mexico.

Length:: about 1.3 m (4 ft).

Colour, markings and features: varied colouration depending on its native region: grey, cream or light-green blotches on the back, which may be olive, brown or black, but also boldly blotched or very dark (in Arizona).

Central and South America

The following dangerous snakes are found in central and South America.

Bushmaster

Habitat: lowland rainforests.

Distribution: lower central America and northern South America.

Length: up to 3 m (10 ft).

Colour, markings and features: light brown, yellowish or tan in colour, with a row of diamond-shaped blotches, sometimes containing two pale triangles, along the back; a dark strip running from the eye to the edge of the mouth.

Cantil

Habitat: dry forests and scrubland.

Distribution: Mexico's western coast.

Length: about 1 m (3 ft).

Colour, markings and features: black or dark brown, with wide bands of paler brown edged with white; a triangular head with a distinctive thin, white line running from the tip of the snout along the upper jaw and another through its eyes.

Eyelash viper

Habitat: trees in tropical rainforests and cloud forests.

Distribution: from southern Mexico to northern Colombia.

Length: about 60 to 70 cm (23 to 27 in).

Colour, markings and features: varied in colour, from uniformly yellow to green with brown blotches or mottled black-and-brown flecks; a cluster of 'eyelashes', or small, spine-like scales, over each eye.

Fer-de-lance

Habitat: moist places near streams and rivers in tropical forests.

Distribution: the northern Amazon basin.

Length: up to 1.5 m (5 ft).

Colour, markings and features: brown or grey; indistinct markings of dark blotches and light streaks, but always with a dark streak running from each eye to the angle of the jaw.

South American coral snake

Habitat: rainforests and plantations.

Distribution: northern South America and the islands of Trinidad and Tobago.

Length: about 1 m (3 ft).

Colour, markings and features: wide, red bands separated by an equally wide combination of black, white, black, white and black bands; the neck is red, with a white bar behind the snout and a black bar passing through the eyes.

South American rattlesnake

Habitat: dry forests, scrub and grassland.

Distribution: from Mexico to Argentina.

Length: about 1.5 m (5 ft).

Colour, markings and features: ranges in colour from light grey through brown, yellow and tan to olive and black; diamonds along the back, usually darker than the background colour and edged in white or yellow; parallel lines on the neck; a warning rattle emanating from the tail if alarmed.

Southern coral snake

Habitat: tropical and cooler forests, farmland and grassland.

Distribution: from central Brazil to southern Argentina.

Length: about 1 m (3 ft).

Colour, markings and features: black, with double white bands, between red bands, so that the sequence is red, black, white, black, white, black, red and so on.

Striped palm viper

Habitat: trees in tropical forests.

Distribution: Costa Rica and Panama.

Length: up to 1 m (3 ft).

Colour, markings and features: the head and body are bluish-green, with some white spots or crossbars on the back; the young are brown, with black-and-white markings, but change to green before assuming adult colouration.

North Africa

The following dangerous snakes are found in North Africa.

Desert black snake

Habitat: deserts, rocky places, parks and wasteground near towns or villages.

Distribution: Egypt, parts of the Arabian peninsula and the Middle East.

Length: about 1 m (3 ft).

Colour, markings and features: usually black or very dark grey; does not spread its hood.

Desert horned viper

Habitat: dunes and wind-blown, sandy regions.

Distribution: North Africa.

Length: about 60 cm (23 in).

Colour, markings and features: sandy, light grey or pinkish in colour, often with a row, or two parallel rows, of darker blotches down the back; a single, long, thorn-like horn over each eye; moves by side-winding; makes a loud, rasping noise when annoyed.

Central Africa

The following dangerous snakes are found in central Africa.

Forest cobra

Habitat: rainforests.

Distribution: tropical and subtropical Africa.

Length: about 2 m (6 ft), but sometimes longer.

Colour, markings and features: the head and front of the body are grey-brown in colour, speckled with black; the lower part of the body is a glossy black; rears up and spreads its narrow hood when alarmed.

Gaboon viper

Habitat: the forest floor.

Distribution: central and eastern Africa.

Length: up to 1.2 m (4 ft).

Colour, markings and features: geometric design of rectangles, triangles and diamonds of cream, purple, pink and various shades of brown, providing excellent camouflage in leaf litter; light and dark lines radiate from the eyes.

Spotted night adder
Habitat: grasslands and lightly wooded areas.
Distribution: central Africa.
Length: about 75 cm (29 in).
Colour, markings and features: grey or greenish, with faint blotches along the back.

East Africa

The following dangerous snakes are found in east Africa.

Green mamba
Habitat: scrub and forests, where it climbs trees.
Distribution: eastern Africa.
Length: about 2 m (6 ft).
Colour, markings and features: a uniform bright green in colour, making it the only plain green snake.

Mozambique spitting cobra
Habitat: grassland and forest clearings.
Distribution: from east Africa to South Africa.
Length: up to about 1.2 m (4 ft).
Colour, markings and features: light grey to olive-brown, with each scale edged in black; yellow or pinkish underneath, with dark crossbars or blotches on the throat; spreads its broad hood and spits venom when alarmed.

Sedge viper
Habitat: rainforests.
Distribution: east and Central Africa.
Length: about 60 cm (23 in).
Colour, markings and features: bright green, with black markings down the back and on the head; the young are dark grey, with few markings apart from a cream tip on the tail; large eyes, with vertical pupils.

West Africa

The following dangerous snakes are found in west Africa.

Carpet (saw-scaled) viper
Habitat: deserts, scrub and dry grassland.
Distribution: west Africa, India and Sri Lanka.
Length: up to 75 cm (29 in).
Colour, markings and features: grey or brown, with a darker area along the centre of the back, in which there are a number of white spots; saw-like scales on the sides make a rasping sound when rubbed together.

Hairy bush viper
Habitat: trees.
Distribution: west Africa.
Length: up to 60 cm (23 in).
Colour, markings and features: usually pale to dark green, but may also be yellowish; spiky, upturned scales.

Rhinoceros viper

Habitat: riverbanks in forested areas.
Distribution: west Africa.
Length: up to 1 m (3 ft).
Colour, markings and features: a row of blue-green, bow-tie-shaped markings, often edged in yellow, on a purple-brown background, with paler-coloured flanks; a cluster of horn-like scales on the snout.

Southern Africa

The following dangerous snakes are found in southern Africa.

African coral snake

Habitat: dry, grassy, rocky and semi-desert areas.
Distribution: western parts of southern Africa, the Cape region and Namibia.
Length: about 50 cm (19 in), but sometimes larger.
Colour, markings and features: orange or pinkish in colour, with black crossbars over the body; red head, with a black line running over it and through the eyes and another black bar on the neck; a large, triangular shield on the snout.

Black mamba

Habitat: grasslands and scrub.
Distribution: southern Africa
Length: up to 2.5 m (8 ft).
Colour, markings and features: despite the snake's name, the body is not actually black, but more dark grey in colour, although the inside of the mouth is black; if threatened, it may spread its narrow hood.

Horned adder

Habitat: scrub, semi-desert and true desert conditions.
Distribution: southern and south-western Africa.
Length: about 40 cm (15 in).
Colour, markings and features: the colour varies according to the habitat and may be grey, tan, reddish or brown; a series of dark blotches runs down the back and there are alternating blotches on each flank; a horn above each eye.

Many-horned adder

Habitat: sandy or rocky places.
Distribution: southern Africa.
Length: about 50 cm (19 in).
Colour, markings and features: grey-brown, with four rows of pale-edged, dark-brown, irregular blotches along the back and dark, pointed markings on the top of the head; clusters of two, three or four horns over each eye.

Peringuey's viper

Habitat: sand dunes.
Distribution: a narrow, coastal strip in the Namib Desert.
Length: up to 1.5 m (5 ft).
Colour, markings and features: light brown, fawn, grey or pinkish in colour, with three rows of faint spots running down the back; a rounded, flattened head, with the eyes set on top, looking straight upwards; moves by side-winding.

Poisons, bites and stings

Rinkhals or spitting cobra

Habitat: grasslands.

Distribution: southern Africa

Length: about 1 m (3 ft).

Colour, markings and features: varied in colour, sometimes black bands on a grey, yellow or orange background, but sometimes plain black or brown; when alarmed, it will rear up and spread its hood.

Throughout Africa

The following dangerous snakes are found throughout Africa.

Boomslang

Habitat: grassland, scrub and light woodland.

Distribution: most of Africa, apart from the Sahara.

Length: about 1.5 m (5 ft), although it can be longer.

Colour, markings and features: females are usually olive-brown; males are various shades of green or blue, with black edges to the scales; when alarmed, it puffs up its throat to display brightly coloured skin between the scales; active by day and a good climber.

Puff adder

Habitat: varied, but not deserts.

Distribution: throughout Africa.

Length: about 1 m (3 ft).

Colour, markings and features: brown or yellowish, with white-edged chevrons on the back.

The Middle East and Asia

The following dangerous snakes are found in the Middle East and Asia.

Indian (spectacled) cobra

Habitat: forests, farmlands and around towns and villages.

Distribution: India, Pakistan and Sri Lanka.

Length: up to 2 m (6 ft).

Colour, markings and features: usually black or dark brown, with lighter markings on the throat; when alarmed, it spreads its very wide hood and may display bold, white markings in the shape of spectacles on the back.

King cobra

Habitat: forests, foothills and cultivated areas.

Distribution: India, southern China, South-east Asia and the Philippines.

Length: up to 5.5 m (28 ft), making it the longest venomous snake in the world.

Colour, markings and features: olive coloured, with black-edged scales; the young are dark brown or black, with chevron-shaped bands of white or yellow; rears up and spreads its narrow hood when alarmed.

Palestine viper

Habitat: dry, sandy areas.

Distribution: the Middle East.

Length: up to 1.3 m (4 ft).

Colour, markings and features: usually grey, light brown or reddish-brown, with a broad, dark-brown or black, wavy-edged line running along the back; two broad, dark lines radiate from the eyes, another crosses the snout.

Pope's pit viper

Habitat: small trees and shrubs in hills and mountain forests.

Distribution: northern India and South-east Asia.

Length: about 90 cm (35 in).

Colour, markings and features: uniformly green, except for the tail, which is red or reddish-brown; young snakes have a pale line, bordered by a red line, running along the flanks (the pale line may be absent in adults); a large, triangular head.

Russell's viper

Habitat: grasslands, scrub and plantations.

Distribution: India, Myanmar (Burma), Pakistan and Sri Lanka.

Length: about 1 m (3 ft), but sometimes longer.

Colour, markings and features: pale greyish-brown, with dark-brown, white-edged ovals on the back, often partly joined together; similar ovals run down the flanks, but alternate with those on the back; wedge-shaped marks radiate from the eyes.

White-lipped pit viper

Habitat: forest trees.

Distribution: north-eastern India to south-eastern China.

Length: about 70 cm (27 in).

Colour, markings and features: a pale-green upper body, but yellow-green underneath; males have a thin, white line running along each side; distinctive orange eyes, with vertical pupils.

South-east Asia

The following dangerous snakes are found in South-east Asia.

Banded krait

Habitat: forests, fields and around houses.

Distribution: throughout South-east Asia.

Length: up to 2 m (6 ft).

Colour, markings and features: alternating black-and-white (or cream) bands of equal width running from the neck to the tip of the tail.

Blue Malayan coral snake

Habitat: forests and agricultural areas.

Distribution: throughout South-east Asia.

Length: up to 1.5 m (5 ft).

Colour, markings and features: head, tail and underside are orange, back is blue-black, sides are pale blue; very shy and rarely seen, but dangerously venomous.

Indonesian spitting cobra

Habitat: forests, farmland and around villages.

Distribution: the Malaysian peninsula and the larger Indonesian islands.

Length: up to 2 m (6ft).

Colour, markings and features: uniformly black, brown or dark grey, with pale areas on the underside of the hood; spits venom.

Poisons, bites and stings

Mangrove snake

Habitat: trees in forests and mangrove swamps.

Distribution: throughout South-east Asia.

Length: up to 1 m (3 ft).

Colour, markings and features: bold, yellow bands on a black background, becoming narrower towards the middle of the back; yellow lips.

Wagler's pit viper

Habitat: dense rainforest, but also found near human habitat, where it lives in trees, so bites often occur on upper body extremeties.

Distribution: Malaysian peninsula and archipelago, Indonesia, Borneo, Philippines.

Length: up to 1 m (3 ft).

Colour, markings and features: green with white cross bands edged with blue or purple. Two dorsal lines on both sides of the head.

Australia

The following dangerous snakes are found in Australia.

Australian coral snake

Habitat: under logs during the day and on then surface at night.

Distribution: eastern parts of Australia.

Length: up to 30 cm (11 in).

Colour, markings and features: pink or red, with irregular crossbars of cream-centred, dark-brown scales; a wide, black band across the head and another on the neck; smooth, shiny scales; a slightly upturned snout; a burrowing snake.

Australian copperhead

Habitat: damp lowlands and highlands.

Distribution: south-eastern Australia and northern Tasmania.

Length: up to 1 m (3 ft), but usually less.

Colour, markings and features: black, dark grey or coppery in colour; smooth scales.

Bandy–bandy

Habitat: forests, grasslands and scrub.

Distribution: most of Australia, apart from the south-west.

Length: up to 60 cm (23 in).

Colour, markings and features: mainly black and white, with about thirty wide, white rings around the body and tail, with the first band passing across the top of the head; a long, slender and smooth body; a burrowing snake, found on the surface at night only.

Black tiger snake

Habitat: rocky places, grass, dunes and beaches.

Distribution: south-western Australia and islands along the southern coast, Tasmania and the islands of Bass Strait.

Length: about 1 m (3 ft), although some islands have dwarf and giant forms.

Colour, markings and features: usually jet black, but occasionally there are traces of lighter crossbands; when alarmed, it may spread its neck, but does not form a hood.

Death adder
Habitat: varied, apart from dry or rocky scrub.
Distribution: found in all parts of Australia, apart from the central desert region.
Length: usually 40 to 50 cm (15 to 19 in), but can measure up to 1 m (3 ft).
Colour, markings and features: varied in colour from grey through brown to red, with irregular crossbands over the body; the tip of the tail is often yellow or cream; a broad, triangular head.

Inland taipan (or fierce) snake
Habitat: dry plains and grasslands.
Distribution: central Australia.
Length: up to 2 m (6 ft).
Colour, markings and features: brown or olive-green, sometimes with black markings scattered over the head, sometimes with a uniformly black head; when alarmed, it may rear up, but does not have a hood.

King brown (or mulga) snake
Habitat: being a very adaptable snake, equally happy in rainforests and deserts.
Distribution: the whole of Australia, apart from the extreme south.
Length: up to 2 m (6 ft).
Colour, markings and features: mid-brown, dark red-brown or dark olive; each scale has a dark border or tip; the colour becomes paler on the sides, and the underside is cream or pinkish in colour; active by day or night, depending on the climate; among the commonest of Australian snakes and dangerously venomous.

Taipan
Habitat: the floor of forests, woodlands and wooded grasslands.
Distribution: north-eastern Australia, the extreme north of Australia and New Guinea.
Length: up to 2 m (6 ft).
Colour, markings and features: light or dark brown, fading to a paler shade at the sides and on the underside; the head is lighter in colour, often cream; active during the day and early evening; shy and secretive, so rarely seen; one of the most dangerously venomous snakes in the world.

Tiger snake
Habitat: forests and open grasslands.
Distribution: south-eastern Australia.
Length: up to 1.2 m (4 ft).
Colour, markings and features: grey, olive or reddish in colour, with a series of lighter-coloured crossbands; when alarmed, it flattens its neck.

Western brown snake
Habitat: varied, from forests to grasslands, plains and deserts.
Distribution: most of Australia, apart from the extreme south-west and south-east.
Length: up to 1.5 m (5 ft).
Colour, markings and features: varied, making identification difficult; can be light

Poisons, bites and stings

brown to black, be a uniform colour or lightly banded around the body, may have a black head and neck or a dark, narrow crossbar; further combinations of these colours and markings are also possible.

Marine snakes

The following dangerous snakes are found in the sea.

Pelagic sea snake

Habitat: tropical and southern waters.

Distribution: from the east coast of Africa to the west coast of central and South America.

Length: up to 1 m (3 ft).

Colour, markings and features: bright yellow, with a dark-brown or black line running along the back; hexagonal scales that do not overlap; a flattened tail and body; may sometimes be washed ashore, but is more often found in enormous shoals in warm seas.

Sea krait

Habitat: reefs, rocky shores and mangrove swamps.

Distribution: around the coasts of India, south-east Asia, the Pacific islands and north-east Australia.

Length: up to 1 m (3 ft).

Colour, markings and features: a yellow-grey snout, alternating black and blue-grey bands of equal width; a flattened tail.

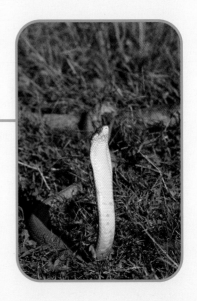

Spider and tick bites

Like snakes, because most venomous spiders do not share our habitats, only a few of the many species of spider in the world are harmful to humans. Some, however, do and are, including the red-back spider and the infamous funnel-web spider. Nevertheless, again like snakes, spiders don't bite unless they have to.

Ticks inhabit most parts of the world, and can even be found in the London parks that are home to herds of deer. Although most tick bites only cause local irritation, some have more serious effects: Lyme disease, whose symptoms resemble those of arthritis, can be caused by deer ticks, for instance, while the venom of other ticks may cause paralysis.

It is important to protect yourself, and your family, from being bitten by spiders or ticks, as follows:
· if you are visiting a country in which there are venomous species, familiarise yourself with their appearance by looking at pictures of them, as well as with their natural habitats, so that you can either avoid these areas or take special precautions when visiting them;
· teach your children to recognise harmful species and to leave them alone;
· if you live in an area that is known to harbour harmful species, regularly clean out any obvious places that may attract them.

The red-back spider
The red-back spider is small and normally black, with a red stripe running along its back. It is found throughout most parts of Australia, in dark spots in which it can live undisturbed, particularly in old tyres, sheds, outhouses and under the eaves of roofs.

Disturbing these spiders can provoke them to bite, most often the hand. The best preventative measure is consequently to wear gloves when cleaning sheds, lifting old tyres or doing any other jobs that may bring you into contact with a red-back spider.

Poisons, bites and stings

The signs and symptoms of a red-back spider bite

The signs and symptoms of a red-back spider bite are as follows:

· feeling a sharp sting;
· localised swelling around the bite;
· pain, firstly at the site of the bite, then more generalised;
· nausea;
· dizziness, and sometimes faintness;
· muscle spasms or weakness;
· profuse sweating;
· a rapid pulse;
· shock (see pages 92 to 94).

Managing a red-back spider bite

Before managing a red-back spider bite:

· assess the scene for danger;
· check the casualty's ABC: airway, breathing and circulation (pulse) (see pages 38 to 41);
· be alert for, and be prepared to treat, the signs of shock (see pages 92 to 94): although these bites can be painful and distressing, they are not necessarily lethal – the associated shock can be more dangerous.

Then take the following steps.

1 Reassure the casualty and seek medical assistance.

2 Apply a cold compress (see page 127) to the area of the bite.

3 Continue to monitor the casualty's ABC until medical assistance arrives.

The funnel-web spider

The funnel-web spider is found in Australia, notably around Sydney, along the coast of New South Wales and in south-eastern Queensland. This black or reddish-brown spider, which measures 2 to 3 cm (to 1 in) in length, is named for the shape of the web that it spins. Although it can be found in rock crevices, post holes, trees and shrubs, it can also make its home underneath houses in both urban and rural locations. For this reason, visitors and residents should be able to identify, and be alert for, the funnel-web spider.

The signs and symptoms of a funnel-web spider bite

The signs and symptoms of a funnel-web spider bite include:

· intense initial pain at the site of the bite;
· nausea and abdominal pain;
· noisy, laboured breathing;
· numbness and muscular weakness;
· profuse sweating;
· drooling saliva emanating from the mouth;
· secretions being coughed up;
· weeping eyes;
· cold skin and shivering.

Managing a funnel-web spider bite

Before managing a funnel-web spider bite:

· assess the scene for danger;
· check the casualty's ABC: airway, breathing and circulation (pulse) (see pages 38 to 41);
· be alert for, and be prepared to treat, the signs of shock (see pages 92 to 94);
· seek medical assistance as a matter of urgency.

Thereafter, do the following.
1 Reassure the casualty and then lay him or her down, with the head and shoulders raised and supported, ensuring that the level of the heart is above that of the wound in order to contain the poison.
2 Wind a wide crêpe or conforming bandage (see page xx), or else a piece of clean fabric or even a pair of nylon tights, over the bite and around the affected limb, as follows:
· apply the bandage firmly enough to compress the tissues, but not so tightly that it restricts the blood flow to the limb below the bandage;
· bandage from the bite to the fingers or toes, then up to the armpit or groin;
· bandage as much of the limb as possible;
· do not remove the bandage after you have applied it.
3 Support and immobilise the affected limb by either applying a splint (see page 139) with a second bandage or padding it with rolled-up blankets or towels.
4 Check the casualty's breathing and circulation again and be prepared to resuscitate (see pages 44 to 53 if necessary. Also look for, and, if necessary, treat, any signs of shock (see pages 92 to 94).

Poisons, bites and stings

Tick bites

Ticks, bloodsucking members of the arachnid (spider) family, are found across the world. They attach themselves to the skin of warm-blooded vertebrates, such as sheep, cattle, deer, dogs and people – with their barbed proboscis. When they've finished feeding, they detach themselves from the source of their meal, then attach themselves to a blade or stem of (often tall) grass and wait for their next meal to pass by. In parklands, it is usually dogs who are plagued by ticks as they snuffle around in the grass; humans rambling through grasslands in shorts can also fall victim to ticks, however.

Although most tick bites do not cause any problems beyond localised skin irritation, if their mouthparts are not carefully removed (see page 235), the bite site may become infected. It is possible to contract Lyme disease from certain ticks, however, while if inflicted in coastal eastern Australia, from Queensland to northern Tasmania, the venom injected by the bite of some ticks can cause paralysis, especially in small children. The tiny ticks responsible are drab in colour, oval and flat in shape – although when their bodies are engorged with blood they may become rounded, measuring about 0.5 cm (¼ in) in diameter – and often hide in body crevices, particularly behind the ears and in the hair, making a careful search advisable.

The signs and symptoms of a tick bite

The signs and symptoms of a tick bite include:
· local irritation around the site of the bite;
· a possible nodule on the skin;
· in severe cases, weakness of the facial muscles and those of upper eyelids, progressing to the arms and chest, sometimes accompanied by breathing difficulties.

If the casualty is a child, or an adult casualty who has not recovered after two hours, it is vital that you seek medical assistance.

Removing a tick

To remove a tick from a casualty's skin, if possible, first apply petroleum jelly or a little alchohol to the tick: this makes it relax its mouthparts. Then slide the open blades of a pair of small, sharp scissors or tweezers over the tick, so that a blade lies on each side of it, and then lever the tick outwards. Ensure that the tick's mouthparts are not left behind.

Injuries caused by marine animals

The best ways of avoiding being injured by marine animals, such as sea urchins, weever fish, bullrouts, stonefish and jellyfish, is to:

· obey all instructions given by lifeguards and notices posted on the beach – if you are asked to leave the water or wear shoes, for example, do so immediately;

· enter the water slowly – don't run or dive in;

· if you feel a sting, back out of the water slowly – don't thrash about because this may prompt whatever stung you to do so again;

· if you are swimming in tropical waters, swim in stinger-resistant enclosures and wear protective swimwear, such as a stinger suit.

· be prepared for stings – carry a supply of household vinegar and broad, conforming bandages (see page 74 o 79);

· if you are rescuing a casualty from the water, take care not be stung yourself.

Managing injuries inflicted by sea urchins

Spiky sea urchins are found in most warm seas, particularly around rocks. Their sharp and brittle spines break off beneath the skin if they are stepped upon or sat on.

Because the spines are so brittle, they must be pulled out in a straight direction. Although it may cause discomfort, a single spine left in the skin will gradually dissolve and disappear without further treatment being required. If many spines are left in the skin, however, seek medical assistance.

Managing injuries inflicted by weever fish

Weever fish, which have sharp, poisonous spines along their backs, are found around the British and continental European coastlines, where they lie close to the shore, half-covered in sand, their spines consequently inflicting injuries to the feet by puncturing the skin, causing swelling and severe pain. Such injuries – especially in children – are easily avoided by wearing beach or 'jelly' sandals, which have thick, flexible soles, when in the water.

If someone is injured by a weever fish, the treatment is straightforward: simply soak the injured foot in a bucket of water as hot as the casualty can bear until the pain eases, which indicates that the poison has been deactivated. You should nevertheless look for, and be prepared to treat, any signs of shock (see pages 92 to 94), especially if the casualty is a child.

Bullrout and stonefish injuries

Skin-penetrating injuries can be caused by the spines of the bullrout and stonefish, both of which are found in tropical inlets, rocky beaches, coral reefs and brackish estuaries. To avoid injury:

· don't pick up a funny-looking rock – it may actually be a bullrout or stonefish;

· don't poke your hand into any rock crevices where these creatures may be lurking;

· wear shoes when walking on rocks and mudflats or wading in rock pools and deep water.

The signs and symptoms of an injury inflicted by a bullrout

The signs and symptoms of an injury inflicted by a bullrout or stonefish are as follows:
· immediate, intense pain at the site of the injury;
· pain spreading from the wound along the affected limb;
· possibly a spine penetrating the wound;
· the injured area may be grey or blue in colour;
· swelling of the injured area;
· irrational behaviour;
· sweating;
· shock (see pages 92 to 94).

Managing an injury inflicted by a bullrout

Before managing an injury inflicted by a bullrout or stonefish:
· assess the scene for danger;
· check the casualty's ABC: airway, breathing and circulation (pulse) (see pages 38 to 41);
· be alert for, and be prepared to treat, the signs of shock (see pages 92 to 94);
· seek medical assistance immediately. Then take the following steps.

1 Reassure the casualty and then, being careful not to scald it, immerse the injured part of the body in hot water until the pain subsides.
2 Remove any foreign body that emerges from the wound.
3 Monitor the casualty's breathing (see pages 39 to 40) and be prepared to administer artificial respiration (see pages 44 to 46).

Jellyfish stings

Most of the jellyfish that are found in temperate waters will inflict painful stings, but these are not generally serious. The only dangerous type of jellyfish found in temperate waters is the Portuguese man-of-war; in tropical waters, bluebottles and box jellyfish are both dangerous.

The signs and symptoms of a jellyfish sting

The signs and symptoms of a jellyfish sting are as follows:

· immediate, intense pain in the part of the body that has been stung;

· whip-like tentacle marks, weals and localised areas of goose pimples (when the sting has been inflicted by a box jellyfish, the marks have a 'frosted-ladder' appearance);

· pain in the chest and abdomen, and sometimes also backache;

· nausea or vomiting;

· a lack of co-ordination in the limbs;

· breathing difficulties and circulation irregularities arising ten to twenty minutes later;

· possibly irrational behaviour;

· shock (see pages 92 to 94).

Managing a jellyfish sting

Before managing a jellyfish sting:

· assess the scene for danger;

· check the casualty's ABC – airway, breathing and circulation (pulse) (see pages 38 to 41) – and be prepared to resuscitate (see pages 44 to 53) if necessary;

· be alert for, and be prepared to treat, the signs of shock (see pages 92 to 94).

Then do the following.

1 Do not rub off the sting, but instead flood the stung area with either vinegar or an alcoholic spirit like gin, vodka or whisky for at least thirty seconds to deactivate the poison and shrivel the stinging tentacles, which can then be brushed off. Now apply a conforming bandage (see pages 74 to 79) to the area.

If no vinegar or alcoholic spirit is available, gently pick off any tentacles with either tweezers or your fingers and then apply a conforming bandage to the area above the sting only.

Do not cease any resuscitation during this time.

2 Monitor the casualty's breathing and circulation and then seek medical assistance as a matter of urgency.

3 Immobilise the affected limb by binding it with bandages. If possible, apply an ice pack (see page 127) to relieve the casualty's pain while you wait for medical help to arrive.

Poisons, bites and stings

Chapter 8

Common sense and accident prevention

Our homes are surprisingly dangerous places: nearly 1.5 million people a year in Britain alone need hospital treatment following accidents in their homes. The most serious domestic injuries are falls, scalds, burns and cuts, all of which can be fatal if the casualty is very young or elderly.

Falls are not only among the most dangerous of all household injuries, but are almost always the most easily avoidable. They often occur as a result of a momentary lapse in concentration, such as when rushing to answer the telephone or doorbell and then tripping over a child's toy, a badly laid carpet or a loose mat. Falls also happen when we stand on unsuitable objects to reach something that is stored high up in a cupboard, to change a light bulb, to clean a window or to paint a wall. Climbing onto a chair is something that we all do, and despite either falling or nearly falling, we continue to do it time after time, thereby unthinkingly putting our lives at risk. Don't become a casualty: use a small set of domestic folding steps, of the type that transform themselves into a stool, for everyday use and a stepladder for larger and higher DIY jobs, making sure that it is fully extended and securely positioned on level ground. And remember: don't overreach yourself when you're up a ladder, but instead climb down and move the ladder to a more suitable position.

Young children are often scalded when, unaware of the danger, they grab objects that older people would never dream of grasping, such as cups of hot drinks, kettles, teapots and toasters – objects that they routinely see their parents using. Keep such objects well out of children's reach, and never spread a tablecloth over the table when toddlers are around because they'll try to hold onto it to pull themselves upright, thereby pulling the things set on it – perhaps things that could burn them – over themselves. Finally, when filling a hot-water bottle, check that it isn't leaking and also that it isn't too hot, and if necessary wrap it in a towel or else use a hot-water bottle that has a protective cover.

Safety checklists 242

Emergency information 250

Safety checklists

Common sense is the most useful tool in your armoury when it comes to accident prevention, so go around your house and identify any changes that need to be made – be it to your home or to your practices – in order to make it a safer place.

Use the following checklists for ideas on how to improve the safety of your home, as well as your and your family's safety when driving, at work or on holiday.

General checklist

Ask yourself the following questions.

· Do you have a first-aid kit? Do you know how to treat an injury and deal with a casualty?

· Do you have any objects in your home, such as a heavy, unstable piece of furniture like a wardrobe or wall mirror, that could cause an injury?

· Are there eye-level markings identifying glass doors, patio doors and French windows?

· Have you checked your electrical equipment, along with flexes and plugs, for wear and tear?

· In case of fire, do you have smoke alarms? For the cost of a few pennies, they could save your family's lives, so if you don't have any smoke alarms in your house, install some. Make sure that they are positioned correctly, that you test them regularly and that either batteries have been fitted or the alarms have been wired into your home's electrical circuit.

· Do you and your family know what to do in the event of a fire? Call the fire brigade; leave the premises without stopping to gather personal items; shut all doors and windows and turn off the electrical power if it is safe to do so; assemble everyone in one place; do not re-enter a burning or smoke-filled house; and do not re-enter your home until the fire brigade tells you that it is safe to do so.

· If you have children, have you inserted dummy plugs into wall sockets to prevent your children from investigating the sockets with their fingers?

Kitchen checklist

Look at your kitchen and ask yourself the following questions.

· Have you arranged any electrical flexes and cords so that they don't trail over the work surfaces n easy reach of children?

· Are any electrical kitchen appliances situated well away from sinks and taps? Water and electricity are a lethal combination.

· Do you turn your saucepan handles inwards, away from the edges of the hob, when they are simmering or boiling? This will prevent you accidentally knocking them over.

· Do you position full teapots, coffeepots and cups of hot drinks away from table edges, and out of reach of young children

· Do you always unplug the kettle before filling it?

· Do you unplug your iron and let it cool down in a safe place before putting it away? A hot iron could set fire to flammable materials.

· Are matches and lighters stored out of the reach of small children?

· Have you stored any dangerous chemicals, such as household bleaches, detergents and oven cleaners, well out of children's reach? (If they are kept under the sink, move them to a less accessible place.)

· Have you stored your kitchen knives safely?

· Have you stored any plastic bags safely and out of reach of young children?

· Do you mop up any spills from the floor to pre-empt slips and falls?

· Is the food in your cupboards, fridge and freezer safe? Is it past its 'use-by' date? Are any tins damaged, rusty or leaking? Are your fridge and freezer set to the correct temperatures? Is chilled, cooked food stored away from raw food? Remember that food presents the worst poisoning risks!

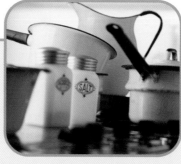

Common sense and accident prevention

Living-room and bedroom checklist

In your living room and bedrooms, ask yourself the following questions.

· Is your furniture made to current safety standards regarding fire hazards? Any upholstered furniture manufactured since 1982 must be labelled if it does not pass the 'match test'.

· Are your family's nightclothes made of non-flammable material?

· Are fireguards positioned in front of any open fires?

· Is a mirror positioned above an open fire? If so, remember that nothing encourages people to lean over a fire more and consider removing it.

· Do you turn off your television and other electrical appliances at night? Unless the appliance is switched off at the socket, the current in the appliance is live.

· Do you close inside doors at night to prevent the spread of smoke and flames in the event of fire?

· If you are a smoker, do you fully extinguish, and safely dispose of, your cigarette or cigar stubs?

· Do you smoke in bed? If so, you are creating a fire hazard.

· Do you switch off your electric blanket before getting into bed? When was the last time you had your electric blanket checked for safety?

· Is there a smoke alarm outside the bedroom door? If not, install one. If so, is it loud enough to wake a sound, deep sleeper? If not, buy a noisier one.

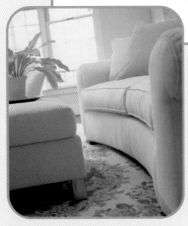
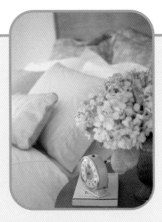

Bathroom checklist

In the bathroom, ask yourself the following questions.
· Has the wiring been professionally fitted and checked? Remember that water and electricity are a lethal combination and never use portable electrical appliances, such as heaters, televisions, radios or hairdryers, in the bathroom. The only permissible electrical plug is a shaver socket. Light switches must either be situated outside the bathroom or be mounted on the ceiling and operated by a pull cord.
· Have you stored any medication out of children's reach?
· Have you returned any unused, or unwanted, medicines to your pharmacist, where they can be disposed of securely and safely?
· Are any scissors or razor blades stored safely out of children's reach?
· Do you check the water temperature before getting into the shower or bath? Do you double-check it before bathing a baby or child? Remember that you must never leave babies or children alone in a bathroom in case they injure themselves, or even drown, so if you must answer the phone or doorbell while bathing a child, wrap him or her in a towel and take him or her with you.
· Are any mats in your bathroom of the non-slip variety?

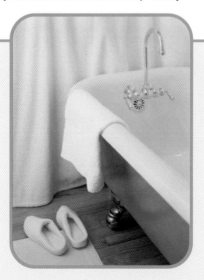

Common sense and accident prevention

Motoring checklist

If you are a driver, ask yourself the following questions.

· Do you have your car serviced regularly? If not, do so.

· Do you check your vehicle before turning on the engine? Do you have four wheels, for instance? Are the tyres inflated to the correct pressure? Are they worn and do they therefore need replacing? Are your lights intact and do they light up when you switch them on? Are your headlights set to the correct position? Is the oil level high enough? Do you have enough fuel for your journey, or else to drive to the nearest service station? Every day we climb into our cars without thinking about such issues, so get into the habit of walking around your car and checking these small details before hitting the road (or another road user!)

· Do you, and all of your passengers, including those in the rear seat, wear a seat belt at all times? If not, do so. If you are the driver, insist that all of your passengers buckle up (we don't argue with airline cabin crew when they tell us to put our seat belts on!)

· Do you check that, if your children are playing outside, they are in full view when reversing your car?

· Do you carry a warning triangle in case your car breaks down? And does your car hold other types of emergency equipment, such as a spare tyre (inflated to the correct

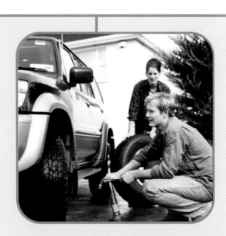

pressure and with the correct amount of tread), fuses and bulbs, a towing rope, a torch, a reflective vest (in case you have to walk on the hard shoulder of the motorway or at night) and a fire extinguisher? If not, consider buying these items.

· Do you drink alcohol before driving? If so, ask yourself whether you would ever let your loved ones be passengers in a car that was being driven by someone who had had a drink.

· Do you drive when you are tired? If so, don't.

· Are all of your documents – your driver's license, insurance and road-worthiness certificate – up to date?

· Is your eyesight good enough to enable you to drive safely? When was the last time you had it checked?

· Do you use a mobile phone when driving? If so, don't, but instead pull over and stop the engine before using the phone.

· Do you comply with the *Highway Code*? Remember the time, energy and money that you spent learning to drive safely, properly and legally. The *Highway Code* comprises a set of laws that must be adhered to, and if you don't, you could cause an accident at worst, and be prosecuted at best.

· Before driving in a foreign country, do you ensure that you know its traffic rules? If not, familiarise yourself with them.

· Have you taught your children road-safety practices, such as how to use and cross roads and how to cycle safely? If not, do so.

Common sense and accident prevention

In the garden

If you have a garden, ask yourself the following questions.
· Do you wear gloves when gardening? If you don't, glass, rusty nails and rose thorns, as well as the sap of some plants, could inflict a serious injury on you.
· Do you store weed-killers, insecticides and fertilisers (even 'natural' organic types) safely and out of the reach of children and pets? If not, do so.
· Do you wear the appropriate clothing and footwear in the garden? Remember never to mow the grass when barefoot or wearing open-toed sandals. Always wear safety goggles when trimming hedges and trees. Before using a chain saw, make sure that you know how to operate it and that you are wearing the correct safety gear.
· Are any ponds, swimming pools or water features in your garden safe? Remember that a child can drown in just a few inches of water.
· Have you made sure that any swimming-pool chemicals are stored correctly and safely?
· When burning bonfires and leaf-waste fires, do you make sure that you are doing so safely and never leave them unattended?
· Are your garden and workshop tools stored correctly? Are any electrically powered tools fitted with circuit-breakers? If not, take the appropriate steps.

At work

If you go to work, ask yourself the following questions.
· Do you, as well as your employer, take safety issues at work seriously?
· Are all of your workmates safety-conscious?
· Do you know who is a trained first-aider?
· Do you know how to evacuate your workplace in an emergency?
If the answer to any of these questions is 'No', take steps to change the situation.

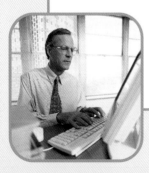

On holiday

Before going on holiday, ask yourself the following questions.

· Are you fully prepared and equipped for your holiday, and have you packed the appropriate clothes? Remember to check with your travel agent and doctor well before your departure date to ensure that you have been given any necessary vaccinations for the country that you will be visiting. The requirements vary from year to year, so even if you have had previous shots, you may still need booster injections.

· Will you be protected from sunburn and insect bites? Remember that even if you will be on the ski slopes, you will still need sun block and sunglasses.

· If you are going on a beach holiday, will you know what the warning flags on the beach mean? Make sure that you understand and obey them, as well as any instructions given by lifeguards.

If you will be sailing, camping, hiking or climbing, ask yourself the following questions and, if necessary, take steps to rectify any negative answers.

· Do you know, and understand, the possible dangers, and have you prepared for them?

· Do you have the correct equipment, such as compasses, matches, maps, torches, clothing and sufficient food and water (stored in secure containers) for everyone travelling with you?

· Do you have all of the necessary safety equipment, such as life jackets, flares, lanterns or a CB radio?

· Do you know how to protect yourself from overexposure to heat or cold?

· Do you know how to signal for help in an emergency?

· Do you know how best to wait for help to arrive if you become lost?

· Will you be with companions? If so, make sure that you stay together.

· Does anyone know where you are going, when you plan to arrive and when you plan to return? If not, give someone the details.

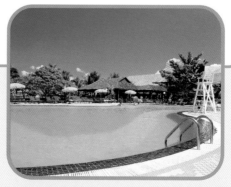

Common sense and accident prevention

Emergency information

Use the following pages to fill in details of your local emergency services and to keep a record of any medication that has been prescribed to members of your family, along with any reactions or allergies from which they may suffer.

Emergency services
Police/fire brigade/ambulance: dial and ask the emergency operator for the relevant emergency service.

Doctor's name:

Surgery's address:

Telephone number:

Surgery hours:

Night service:
Telephone number:

Hospital's name:

Address:

Telephone number:

Dentist's name:

Surgery's address:

Telephone number:

Surgery hours:

Local gas emergency service telephone number:

Common sense and accident prevention

People to contact in an emergency

Name:

Address:

Telephone number (home):

Telephone number (work):

Name:

Address:

Telephone number (home):

Telephone number (work):

List of medications and allergies

Fill in this list for each member of your family, giving details of any medications taken, any allergies suffered, for example, to nuts or penicillin, and any reactions to medications.

Name: **Name of medicine**   **Allergies/reactions**

Name: **Name of medicine**   **Allergies/reactions**

Name: **Name of medicine**   **Allergies/reactions**

Name: **Name of medicine**   **Allergies/reactions**

Name: **Name of medicine**   **Allergies/reactions**

Common sense and accident prevention

Index

After word

A number of international organizations exist to train first-aiders.

The **St John Ambulance** offers training courses to suit all ages and at a range of levels from beginners to more advanced first aid techniques. You will find them in your telephone book, or check out their website for their calendar of training sessions near you. www.sja.org.uk

Other institutions such as the **Red Cross** (and its sister organization the Red Crescent) offer similar training courses. Your local swimming pool or leisure centre may also offer life-saving sessions, so check these out too.

For information and training for first-aides in the workplace, contact the **Health and Safety Executive** (UK) or your local Occupational Workplace Safety Office for advice.

National and international motoring organizations will provide advice on safe motoring at home and abroad, and will inform of individual country's requirements regarding the type of first aid kit required.

Your **local Fire Prevention Officer** (look in your phone book under Fire Prevention) will be able to help to offer advice on fire safety in the home and workplace.

In all emergencies, make sure you know how to call for help. Do not delay in asking for qualified medical assistance from the emergency services at any time.